W9-BRT-033

Swim Your Way to Fitness

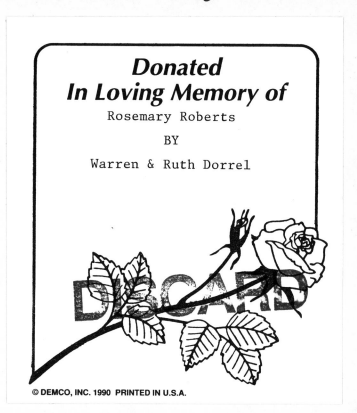

**Donated
In Loving Memory of**
Rosemary Roberts

BY

Warren & Ruth Dorrel

© DEMCO, INC. 1990 PRINTED IN U.S.A.

DISCARD

DISCARD

DISCARD

Swim Your Way to Fitness

A Lifetime of Exercise Programs

Joseph E. McEvoy, D.P.E.

SHELBYVILLE-SHELBY COUNTY
PUBLIC LIBRARY

STACKPOLE
BOOKS

098201

Copyright © 1993 by Stackpole Books

Published by
STACKPOLE BOOKS
5067 Ritter Road
Mechanicsburg, PA 17055

All rights reserved, including the right to reproduce this book
or portions thereof in any form or by any means, electronic or
mechanical, including photocopying, recording, or by any
information storage and retrieval system, without permission in
writing from the publisher. All inquiries should be addressed to
Stackpole Books, 5067 Ritter Road, Mechanicsburg, PA 17055.

A different version of this book was previously published as *Fitness Swimming—
Lifetime Programs* (1985).

Printed in the United States of America

Illustrations by Kim Ruehle Dickerson and Kim Banister
Cover photo by John Foster
Swimmer: Matt Stanek
Cover design by Mark Olszewski
First Edition
10 9 8 7 6 5 4 3 2 1

Library of Congress Cataloging-in-Publication Data

McEvoy, Joseph E.
   Swim your way to fitness : a lifetime of exercise programs /
Joseph E. McEvoy.
     p.   cm.
   ISBN 0-8117-3090-5
   1. Swimming. 2. Exercise I. Title.
GV837.M394   1993
613.7'16—dc20
                                    93-28210
                                       CIP

Dedicated to my wife, Pat,
who has coached the coach and
taught the teacher so many things
over the past twenty-four years.

In 1954 my parents pledged $35 in
seven $5 installments toward the construction of
a municipal swimming pool in Livingston, New Jersey.
It's amazing to think where that
small investment has led me . . .

Contents

Foreword

HABITS ARE HARD to break, so it was a long time before I gave up merely chattering about how nice it would be to swim during the noon hour and actually went trudging over to the college pool. It was an intimidating experience. The pool was open to adult swimmers for only brief periods each day, and then only if a lifeguard remembered to show up. I could manage a dozen lengths or so if I stayed with the side stroke and the elementary back stroke, but the crawl was a killer. Worse yet, no one seemed to care when I triumphantly swam two lengths without stopping. So it was not surprising that I quit swimming after a couple of weeks.

It was two more years before I found my way back to the gym and into the pool. This time, at least, I had three friends with me. We still had plenty of problems—aching muscles we didn't know we had, water in the ear and up the nose, and wet towels steaming up the locker—and swimming was still basically a discouraging experience. We didn't seem to accomplish anything, despite our efforts, and a vague disquiet gradually replaced our hopes for fun in the water.

Then one day Joe McEvoy appeared. As if by magic, the college pool was open for as long each day as the library. Lifeguards were always on time. A friendly voice could be counted on to give encouragement, to suggest an improvement here or there, to hint at fresh possibilities, and to set our aspirations higher. I still remember the day I was told flat out to swim twenty lengths. I'd never done more than four at a time before then, although I harbored a secret goal of doing ten in a row. But Coach Joe said twenty, so why not? And I survived to brag about it for days afterward.

We now have a full-fledged and excitingly varied program for adult lap-swimmers. This book describes the steps by which each of us was led from an initial knock on McEvoy's door to a level of involvement that could become as rigorous as Masters-level competition but that most certainly included membership in Joe's famous Fitness Swimming Club. The adults who regularly dip their toes in our pool come from all walks of life: college faculty and staff, business and professional people from the town, homemakers, retired folk, students from the law school. Some are in the water at 6:00 each morning and others swim only at night, but the most popular time is the noon hour.

I'm a noon-hour type myself, and I've got lots of comrades now and lots of camaraderie. Our motivation is always the same: Swimming laps is good for us. Our bodies like the exercise and we like each other's company. Our emotions are cooled by the rhythmic relaxation, our thoughts are allowed to wander creatively, and our drive for accomplishment is given a pleasing outlet. Even the walk to the gym is an opportunity to wind down from the morning's tensions and warm up one's muscles in preparation for the day's workout.

Swimming laps illustrates the important truth that education is a lifelong adventure, that it is deeply satisfying to perfect old skills and acquire new ones. The standards of excellence in swimming are a blend of individualized self-surpassing goals and general goals appropriate to all people of similar age or ability. Thus there is something marvelously democratic about a swimming pool. When everyone is dressed in a swimsuit it is hard to be pretentious or to pull rank. People who excel in one aspect of swimming meet others whose achievements lie in some other aspect,

and there is plenty for each one to learn from everyone else. Swimming also requires total involvement. In the water, enjoying your harmony with its buoyancy, using its resistance to propel yourself forward, you are no longer fragmented into mind and body, thinker and doer. You discover yourself as someone who at once thinks, feels, wills, and acts.

Like the library, the swimming pool is a resource for those who wish to be educated, who seek life's fullness by enlarging their awareness of the world's possibilities and their own capacities. Coach Joe's book is a guided tour through that library. Read it with caution, because if you stay with it to the end, you will be hooked on swimming for the rest of your life. Eventually, if you don't watch out, you will begin to grow webbing between the toes.

When my friends and I had at long last swum the required 100 miles, we were eligible to become full-fledged members of the Fitness Swimming Club. We celebrated on the outdoor patio beside the pool by festooning a crate with tablecloth and candelabrum. Champagne and caviar were served, in celebration of our transmogrification from mere water churners into bona fide lap swimmers. A couple of years later, several of us contracted to "swim the English Channel" over the semester break. Each half mile or mile we logged in the pool was translated onto a huge wall chart monitoring our progress from Dover to Calais. We urged each other on, warning about ships and jellyfish and other swimmers, noting when the white cliffs could no longer be seen and when the rocks of Cape Gris-Nez were first sighted. We commemorated everyone's completion of the 21-mile swim by preparing a full-

course French dinner, lacking only truf-
fles to give it a five-star rating.

Such fantasies and their celebration
may seem mere foolishness, but they are
at the same time profound occasions. In
such play we celebrate the wonder of
being human. In our aquatic recreation
we prepare ourselves for the deeper tri-
umphs and challenges of life. I can't
imagine a better way to spend an hour
each day. I hope you will soon be joining
us.

George Allan
Dean of the College
Dickinson College

Preface

THERE IS MORE to swimming for fitness than just jumping into the pool and doing some laps. The need for more variety when doing the same kinds of things on a regular basis is a continuing problem for people who exercise several days a week, regardless of their sport. This book is designed as a comprehensive source for those who would like to use swimming as a fitness activity. It describes the options available for fitness swimming to help you remain involved with this activity. It builds on sixteen years of field testing with a wide variety of college-age and adult fitness swimmers. *Swim Your Way to Fitness* blends what fitness swimmers actually do in the pool and what they could do or ought to try.

I was first exposed to the idea of swimming for fitness in the early 1960s as a lifeguard and water safety instructor. Each summer a huge chart would be posted in the pool office at Memorial Pool in Livingston, New Jersey, and some of the regular patrons would complete 50 miles in the American Red Cross Swim and Stay Fit program. At the time, the distance seemed impossibly long, and the whole idea seemed crazy to me. I thought it was funny to watch someone do a "cannonball" by the side of one of these lap swimmers, and then swim away quickly underwater, having interrupted the lap swimmer's workout for the tenth time that day. I really didn't understand what these lap swimmers were doing.

As a freshman at Springfield College in 1965–66, I first read about swimming for fitness (one of the areas of expression in swimming) and organic condition (one of the factors that control success in swimming) in the 1960 edition of Charles E. Silvia's *Manual for Swimming, Water Stunts, Diving, Lifesaving, and Water Safety* (pp. 4–5). This manual accompanied the basic swimming course and was the start of my aquatics education there. I began to understand more about swimming being the "best" exercise, but it would be eleven more years before I tried it myself and began to prepare notes for my first book about fitness swimming.

A landmark publication for me was Kenneth Cooper's *Aerobics* (1968), which, although it emphasized jogging and running (but included some swimming), marked a transition in physical fitness from a strength orientation to a cardiovascular orientation (in other words, it's better to have a healthy heart than big biceps). Cooper explained exercise theory in popular terms and directed people into planned, progressive training programs. It was an important step forward when the average person began talking about cardiovascular conditioning, training effects, heart rates, 12-minute tests, and 30 points a week. Yet I remember wondering why those who ran well and were models of aerobic fitness didn't always do so well in the swimming pool.

I completed valuable apprenticeships in aquatics at Springfield College from 1965 to 1975 and at Pine Knoll Swim School in Springfield, Massachusetts, from 1970 to 1975. The principal guidance in my aquatics education was provided by Professor Silvia, the swimming coach at the college and the director of the summer swim school. This educational environment provided my first exposure to fundamental teaching procedures and to virtually all aspects of competitive swimming. Most importantly, Coach Silvia was a master of stroke technique with a unique approach to the understanding of highly skilled performance. He described the stroke movements of swimming in mechanical, kinesiological, and anatomical terms.

I began my own personal fitness swimming program and started to prepare my first book, *Fitness Swimming—Lifetime Programs* (published in 1985 by Princeton Book Company), in 1976 while teaching at the University of Georgia. The original fitness swimming course was designed in 1976–77 as a parallel to the jogging course there and was first taught in 1978. High enrollments and positive student reactions made it obvious that this course was a good addition to the basic physical education program and that fitness swimming was a vast, untapped market for teachers and students.

When I started teaching at Dickinson College in 1979, I encountered an eager group of faculty swimmers whose enthusiasm led to the establishment of our Fitness Swimming Club and Fitness Swimming Hotline. The course in fitness swimming has run the gamut from conventional scheduling (such as Monday, Wednesday, Friday from 2:00 to 2:50 P.M.) to independent study with up to 100 hours a week available to complete the requirements.

It has been exciting to see the field of fitness swimming taking shape and form. But there is still a long way to go to catch up with the area of fitness running. There seems to be a substance of common knowledge shared by most runners, but swimmers haven't yet developed this body of knowledge within their group. Runners seem more knowledgeable about their equipment, the details of exercise physiology, the basic anatomy of their muscles and joints, and different kinds of training systems.

On the other hand, swimmers as a group do some very good things for themselves. They seem to train more sensibly and to be less abusive to their bodies than runners, and consequently they suffer very few injuries in the pool. Without the lure of a marathon, swimmers think less about increasing mileage or yardage. There is less hurting during the activity and less awareness of "hurt, pain, agony" barriers to surmount. Swimmers seem to be more time-efficient in their training and to grasp the concept that "less is more." There is little confusion between fitness goals (99 percent of all participants) and competitive goals (Masters swimmers).

I have been working in fitness swimming curriculum development since 1976, and this field still feels new and fresh to me. My interest in this area grows out of teaching and helping students, faculty, and townspeople to use swimming as a lifelong form of exercise. The challenge in writing a book such as this is to capture the content of our classes and informal teaching within its pages in order to share this message with a wider audience—namely, you. I sincerely believe that fitness swimming is a great way to exercise and hope that you can enjoy this approach to it for the rest of your life!

ONE

Fitness Swimming

SWIMMING IS ONE of the very best forms of exercise because it permits total body movement in a highly cushioned environment (the water). It's a nearly perfect example of a low-impact or soft-impact aerobic activity, with low risk of injury.

Fitness swimming is a planned program of lap swimming that taps into the tremendous variety inherent in the activity for a lifetime of physical fitness. You can't find a better path to fitness than back and forth in your lap lane.

Water is a unique medium in which to exercise because of the following:

• Buoyancy greatly reduces weight-bearing stress on joints and muscles.

• The water resists movement so that the swimmer exercises with relatively slow movements and slow total body velocity.

• The swimmer's usual horizontal position assists in returning blood to the heart during activity.

• The temperature and high conductivity of water help to remove heat from the body during exercise.

PHYSIOLOGICAL ASPECTS OF SWIMMING. Fitness swimming will provide you with many physical benefits. Here are some of the things that exercise, and swimming in particular, can and cannot do for you:

Cardiac, respiratory, and vascular systems. Regular lap swimming will bring your heart, lungs, and blood vessels to higher levels of efficiency to pump your blood, provide oxygen to working muscles, and remove waste products.

Muscular endurance. As you push and pull your body weight through the water, you will especially develop your muscular endurance—the ability to apply submaximal force over and over again. Swimmers' muscles are not the bulging muscles of a bodybuilder; rather, they will develop to carry you through lap after lap in the pool. The repetitive nature of the arm and leg movements in swimming primarily involves this factor of muscular endurance rather than pure muscular strength. Swimming movements are repeated hundreds

1

of times in an average fitness swimming workout.

Flexibility. The slow, gentle, rhythmic movements of swimming promote joint and muscular flexibility—the ability of your joints to operate painlessly with great freedom of motion and no restrictions. Your warm-up stretching exercises before you swim will also help develop this quality.

Weight control. You can gain some control over your percent body fat (the portion of your body weight that consists of fat) through frequent exercise. You may experience weight loss if you combine exercise with dietary and lifestyle changes. At this point, simply understand that you'll burn extra calories every time you swim laps.

Heart disease prevention. Many factors make an individual more susceptible to heart disease, including high blood pressure, being overweight, smoking, diet and food intake, lack of exercise, and heredity. Some of these factors are controllable, but much depends on when you begin to control them and to what extent, how much damage has already been done, and what is the relative influence of the less controllable factors. There is no system of exercise (or medicine or surgery) that can absolutely guarantee immunity from a heart attack. Claims of this type are false and play on deep-seated fears that motivate some people to exercise. Exercise does promote the development of collateral circulation around and within the heart muscle itself, and this additional blood supply can significantly improve a heart attack victim's chances of survival and recovery.

Longevity. Another hopeful myth connects exercise with long life. This re-

lationship is suggested but not certain, and we all know of too many exceptions to make this a general rule. Many factors blend together to determine our life span, and exercise is one of them, but it is certainly not the whole picture. This relationship is clarified by the saying "While exercise may not add years to your life, it will add life to your years."

To create these desirable "training effects," you must exercise long enough (duration), hard enough (intensity), often enough (frequency), and in different ways (variety).

PSYCHOLOGICAL ASPECTS OF SWIMMING. Beyond the physiological factors, exercise provides psychological benefits and incentives for many participants:

Enjoyment. Fitness swimming is fun. Try to exercise with a joyful and playful spirit, with a sense of wonder about your physical capabilities, and with gratitude that you are alive and active. Get away from the idea of exercise as drudgery, daily duty, or punishment. Find the joy in enjoyment.

Feeling good. Most people feel better when involved in a regular exercise routine. You'll be more alert and have more energy every day. Because this effect is not long lasting, it can provide a strong incentive to exercise frequently. To some, this benefit is justification enough for participation in fitness swimming. These individuals regard any physiological benefits simply as bonuses above and beyond this primary factor of feeling good.

Accomplishment. Learning new skills, developing your stamina, and challenging your present abilities with short-term and long-range goals can make a positive contribution to your self-image and self-confidence. Test your physical and mental limits with a challenging and varied fitness swimming training program.

Change of pace. Fitness swimming can provide a pleasant change from your regular daily routine. Most fitness swimmers return to normal responsibilities with a refreshed and invigorated attitude after exercising. But be sure to leave your problems outside the pool, or they'll ruin your swim workout as well.

Tension reduction. Because we can't always fight or run away from stressful situations, our bodies' reactions to stress are frequently blocked. Exercise can provide a release from physical and emotional tensions, such as anxiety, depression, or unexpressed anger, by using normal stress responses in big-muscle activity and total-body movement. This is also a temporary effect, and tensions may build up again before the next time you swim.

Isolation. Fitness swimming can be a very private and personal time. No one can talk to you; you're on your own in a sensory-deprived environment. This is something you do for yourself and by yourself. You're completely self-reliant in the water.

"Swimmer's high." Occasionally you may experience a heightened sense of well-being while swimming, a feeling that you and the activity blend together with no apparent effort and that you are in perfect harmony with the water rather than struggling against it. You are focused, centered, and absorbed in the activity, altering your normal senses of time, speed, space, and self. You can't force this to happen. It won't occur every time you swim, but it's a terrific sensation when you're in the "flow."

Exercise addiction. For a few people, these psychological benefits become abnormally important, and they become "addicted" to exercise. Exercise dominates their lifestyle, becoming more important than their work, family, and social activities. They may work out two or three times a day. They suffer delusions of invincibility, ignoring serious injuries and disregarding advice to slow down or stop. When deprived of exercise, they experience withdrawal-type symptoms. Denial of this problem is common, and in these cases some type of psychological counseling is needed.

REQUIREMENTS FOR FITNESS SWIMMING. Fitness swimming appeals to people with different levels of involvement and interest. The basic requirements are as follows:

Knowledge. This factor consists mostly of your understanding of what to do, how to do it, and how to keep it interesting, plus the application of some very basic exercise principles to your daily workouts.

Skill. While some skill in strokes, breathing, and turns is required, you do not have to be a championship swimmer to get exercise benefits from fitness swimming. Most fitness swimmers are average swimmers.

Attitude. You must have a desire to learn, a willingness to challenge yourself, and the ability to tolerate some initial discomfort and to reject the many excuses often used to stay out of the water.

In any pool where people swim for fitness, a wide range of these factors is seen. Some swimmers are tremendously knowledgeable and well read about swimming and exercise theory. Others think hand paddles go on their feet. Some are extremely skillful with fancy strokes and flip turns, and they have a different swimsuit for each day of the week. Others swim mostly the crawl stroke, frequently get water up their noses, choke loudly and conspicuously, and try something different only when they think no one is watching. Some are so into swimming that they actually suffer from mental depression if they can't swim eight times a week. The dedication of others reflects less than a lifetime commitment to exercise.

When you are just starting out, you may be especially susceptible to negative influences. You may feel foolish or out of place or that your present skill level is inadequate and will never improve. You may feel intimidated by other swimmers or think that others are watching you. You may feel that no one else has ever been as inept as you are when you swim. You may suffer humilia-tion, embarrassment, and physical distress when you swim, and you may want to drop out.

Remember—you're not the first one to try this, you are not alone in your efforts, and you are not the worst swimmer of all time. My experience with hundreds of beginning fitness swimmers has been that the first one to two weeks may be a little shaky and cautious, but by weeks two to four you'll begin to condition and grow more confident. You'll be amazed with yourself by weeks four to six if you'll just stick with it. You will almost feel yourself getting better from workout to workout and from week to week.

It is estimated that there are 20 million to 60 million fitness swimmers in this country. And there's always room for one more swimmer in our fitness lane—especially if it's you!

TWO

Basic Exercise Theory

THIS CHAPTER PRESENTS some practical applications of basic exercise theory as well as other factors you must consider as you get started in fitness swimming.

Medical Check

Discuss your exercise plans with a physician before you begin a training program, especially if you're over thirty years of age. There are some medical conditions that place limitations on exercise and that require monitoring by a physician. So consult your doctor and start safely.

Gradual Start

It is important to start your fitness-swimming program gradually to let yourself condition over a period of time and to establish the groundwork for lifetime participation. The long-term effects of inactivity cannot be reversed quickly, and regular, enjoyable, and sustained exercise is required to achieve desirable results.

One problem in all exercise programs is that many people start out with a great burst of enthusiasm and resolution, expend their energy much too quickly, and then drop out of the program after a relatively short time. Some fitness swimmers are too vigorous and too competitive, working too hard too soon, then leaving the program without achieving any of the long-range benefits. Start slowly, build up gradually, and stay with the program for the rest of your life.

Frequency of Exercise

Frequency refers to the number of times per week that you exercise. Some fitness swimmers swim seven days a week, and others once every week or two. Three days a week would be a good starting point, and is the required minimum for our Fitness Swimming Course here.

Most fitness swimmers participate three to five times per week, and this is a good range for achieving exercise benefits and training effects. I like to exercise on Monday, Tuesday, Thursday, and Friday, occasionally doing something extra on Wednesdays or over the weekend.

Duration of Exercise

Duration refers to the length of each workout. A good range here would be 15 to 45 minutes per swim, with 30 minutes being about average.

Building up your exercise times and distances progressively is an important part of getting started. But many swimmers ultimately reach a point where they can swim for several hours nonstop. After months of fitness swimming, the duration question will become, How much time do I want to put into my swim today? I like to do a lot of half-hour swims, randomly mixing strokes, pulls, kicks, and other training procedures.

Although exercise tolerance varies widely, any additional fitness benefits that might occur from workouts longer than an hour do not compare favorably with the time and effort invested.

Some factors influencing duration of workouts include availability and convenience of the facility, fitness goals, present level of conditioning, outside demands and pressures, level of energy and enthusiasm, and enjoyment and satisfaction derived.

Some swimmers use a "cycle" method of training, in which long, hard workout days are alternated with days of shorter, quicker, and easier workouts. Weekly or even monthly cycles can be created.

Never punish yourself with exercise. Always try to feel good about your workouts and training program even though you may experience some normal discomforts as you work toward your fitness goals. Positive feelings about your exercise program will help you work long enough and regularly enough to reach and maintain the desired long-term fitness benefits.

Intensity of Exercise

To create training effects from exercise, fitness swimmers must work out within a certain range of intensity. The formula below uses heart rate as the indicator of how hard you are working. Heart rate is directly related to aerobic capacity (a more sophisticated measure of exercise intensity but less practical to use), and you usually reach your maximum heart rate and aerobic limits at the same time.

Individuals' heart rate responses to exercise vary, but individual characteristics and differences are not usually accounted for in standard formulas. Fitness swimmers should develop a sensitivity to their personal reactions to their workouts and training programs ("perceived effort") and should not become obsessively concerned with some arbitrary standards.

The method of determining intensity used in this book requires that you work out at 60 to 80 percent of your maximum heart rate. Your maximum heart rate (beats per minute) can be estimated by subtracting your age from 220. Multiply this maximum heart rate by .60 and .80 to determine the range of intensity. For example: 220 (standard) − 44 (age) = 176 (maximum) x .80 = 140 beats per minute during exercise and 220 − 44 = 176 x .60 = 105 beats per minute during exercise.

This fitness swimmer should try to

swim at a speed or pace that will maintain his or her heart rate on average between 105 and 140 beats per minute throughout the workout.

You may want to adjust the above formula down by 10 to reflect the fact that your maximum heart rate and exercising heart rate each tend to be about 10 beats slower while swimming than for comparable exertion on land, mostly because of your horizontal position in the water.

Count your heart rate once or twice during your workout and again at the end. Using a pace clock or watch, count the number of beats for 6 seconds; then multiply that count by 10 to get your heart rate in beats per minute. Take your heart rate at the carotid artery, the pulse of which can be felt at the side of the throat. Use light pressure, and count immediately when you stop swimming. Even a brief delay can reduce the count.

Check your heart rate frequently when first starting your fitness-swimming program to ensure that you're working within a safe intensity range. After months and years of participation, you should still check your heart rate, but you will need to do so less frequently because you'll know you're within your target heart rate range by how you "feel" as you swim.

The basic problem in exercise intensity is determining a level of exertion that will lead to fitness benefits and improvements without exhausting yourself. Practical intensity levels are: 100 to 140 beats per minute for older people or unconditioned participants, and 120 to 160 for young adults and well-conditioned swimmers.

Intensity levels may change in different workouts or within the same workout. These heart rate guidelines represent averages, not absolutes, and should not be rigidly interpreted or applied. Doing *some* exercise is certainly better than doing no exercise at all.

Caloric Expenditure

Many people start exercise programs with the goal of weight reduction. When you swim, you will burn approximately 10 calories per minute, or 600 calories per hour. Since most people work out on average for 30 minutes, they use up about 300 calories in most of their workouts. In order to lose 1 pound of body weight, you must burn 3,500 calories. As most fitness swimmers swim three to four times a week, it would take at least three weeks of fitness swimming to achieve this weight loss.

The combination of exercise and sensible nutrition gives the best results for weight loss. But it's difficult for some to change the way they eat, what they eat, and how much they eat. And those calories burned up through exercise are all too easily replaced in the form of snacks throughout the day or larger portions during meals.

There is no special food or diet plan that could be fairly presented as being ideal for swimming, particularly in the realm of fitness. There are hundreds of diet books available, all with staunch advocates and followers. Unfortunately, many of them present totally conflicting ideas and advice. Because people are different and have different metabolisms, different diets may work well for different people. Common to all successful plans are self-discipline, willpower, and good sense about food intake.

Weight loss should be gradual, perhaps 1 to 2 pounds per week for most people. It is important to avoid the "yo-yo effect": a steady cycle of being on a diet and losing weight alternated with being off the diet and regaining the weight. And remember that you are not likely to change your total personality, temperament, and body type just by reorganizing your eating habits.

Clearly, exercising more and eating less is important for weight control and reduction, but it is just a starting point. If losing weight is very important to you, you'll need to learn more from other sources about sensible nutrition and diet.

Planning

Fitness swimmers should plan their workouts in advance and then carry them out as planned. This planning helps to build anticipation and enthusiasm, and the follow-through to comple tion gives a sense of accomplishment. You may plan from day to day, on a weekly basis, or even for several weeks into the future in terms of training goals and ideas. You should rarely change a workout in the middle of doing it; this makes your workout too subject to whim and transient feelings of fatigue. Challenge yourself—finish what you've set out to do.

Some workouts have a "balanced" emphasis, featuring several different strokes or procedures, while others have a "focused" emphasis, concentrating on one particular stroke or procedure. A few workouts fall in between these two types, perhaps varying a focused emphasis slightly but not enough to create a truly balanced effect. In your planning, you must answer the following questions:

• Which method of training will you use: continuous swimming or swim and rest, swim and rest . . . ?

• Which workout format will you use: lap swimming or swimming for a time period?

• How much time do you have to plan your workout?

• What symbols should you use to write down the workout?

• What total distance or time period do you wish to complete?

• Will your workout be balanced, focused, or in between?

• What will be the components of the various sets and subsets?

• How much will you warm up before your workout and how much will you warm down afterward?

• How much will you work on your strengths and how much on your weaknesses?

Keeping a Diary

Some very serious swimmers keep records or diaries of their daily programs, including workouts, swimming times, special variations in the workout, body weight, health problems, total distances, stroke problems and corrections, future goals, new ideas, subjective feelings about the workout, and personal items. It's a way to summarize an important part of your lifestyle, to become more thoughtful about your training program, and to compare your present status with what you've done in the past.

Breaks in Training

Don't feel pressured into swimming every day all year round if you feel you need a break. Short breaks from training help to alleviate the boredom and monotony that can set in from doing the same activity over and over. During these breaks, if your goal is fitness for life, pursue other aerobic activities, and be sure to get sufficient rest and relaxation. When you return to fitness swimming, be sure to start in slowly and build back up gradually.

Before and After You Swim

Never suddenly start or stop exercising hard—always ease your way into the activity, and always ease your way back out of the activity. Always prepare your heart, lungs, muscles, and joints for exercise, and always allow these systems to return to a more normal state before you finish your workout. Even though fitness swimming is a low-impact or soft-impact aerobic activity and your chances of injury or sudden death are remote, you will feel better if you incorporate these procedures into each of your workouts.

If possible, walk to the pool. This may be the best warm-up of all. If you do drive, park at the end of the parking lot farthest from the swimming facility so that you will have a longer walk.

Spend 2 to 3 minutes doing some stretching and flexibility exercises before you get in the pool to swim. These form a "general warm-up," suitable not only for swimming but for other sports as well. There are many exercises you can do. I like the following:

• Stand 4 to 5 feet from a wall (or a pool ladder or starting block) and place your hands against it at about shoulder level. Lean into the wall with your body straight, one leg forward (knee bent), and the other leg back (knee straight). Keep the heel of the back leg on the ground to stretch the back of your lower leg. Hold for 8 to 10 seconds, then switch legs.

• Stand 4 to 5 feet from a wall and place your hands against it at about shoulder level. Keeping your arms straight, bend forward and drop your head down lower than your shoulders. Hold for 8 to 10 seconds.

• Brace yourself with one hand against a wall. Stand on your left foot, bend the other knee, and grasp your right foot behind you with your right hand. Pull your foot up and back as you bend forward very slightly to stretch the front of your leg. Hold for 8 to 10 seconds. Repeat for the other leg.

• Grasp a pool ladder or starting block with your arms straight, keeping your feet on the ground directly below your hands. Move your hips back and down to stretch in a semipike position. Hold for 8 to 10 seconds.

• Circle one arm backward as if doing a one-arm back stroke. Do 8 to 10 repetitions. Repeat for the other arm.

• Circle one arm forward as if doing a one-arm crawl stroke. Do 8 to 10 repetitions. Repeat for the other arm.

• Circle one arm forward and one arm backward at the same time. Do 8 to 10 repetitions. Repeat in the opposite direction. Gotcha!!—but this can be done.

• Swing your arms from side to side parallel to the ground, crossing them in front of your body and stretching them back as far as possible behind your body. Do 8 to 10 repetitions.

• Swing your arms up and down vertically in front of yourself. Start back behind your hips, and then swing up to a full reach high above your head. Do 8 to 10 repetitions.

• Join your hands over your head with your elbows bent and with your arms just behind your head. Stretch both arms to the right side as far as possible, and then stretch back to the left side as far as possible. Lean a little to each side as you stretch. Hold each way for 8 to 10 seconds.

• Hang from a chinning bar with your

hands at shoulder width. Stretch from your hands and arms right down through your toes. Sink down between your arms so that your shoulders move up by your ears. Hold for 8 to 10 seconds.

• Once you get down in the water, lean back against the pool wall. While keeping your back against the wall, stand on one leg, grasp your other knee, and pull it up to your chest and shoulder. Hold for 8 to 10 seconds. Repeat for the other leg.

Stretch in the locker room if you're self-conscious about doing these warm-up exercises out on the pool deck. Always stretch smoothly and gently, never using sudden or jerky movements. Be very careful about slipping with wet feet on slippery pool decks. Extremes in flexibility are not needed by most fitness swimmers, and many programs overemphasize these types of exercises, although older fitness swimmers may want to do much more stretching, as joint and muscular flexibility declines with age.

Once in the pool, do not swim fast right away. The first 5 to 10 percent of your total lengths should be very slow, using easy swimming, pulling, kicking, or a combination of these in what is known as a "specific warm-up" (warming up for swimming by swimming very slowly).

Note that whether or not a warm-up is written into the sample workouts in this book, you are advised to complete some type of general and specific warm-up procedures before your swimming workout. If a sample workout doesn't include a warm-up, add several lengths on at the beginning of the workout as a very slow warm-up, or use the first few lengths of the written workout as the warm-up period before swimming faster.

For fitness swimming, you need at least two speeds in the water—one very slow, barely moving for your warm-ups and warm-downs, and the other a little faster, the more normal swimming speed for the main part of your swimming workouts.

The last 2 to 5 percent of your total lengths should be devoted to warming down. These should also be very slow, using easy swimming, pulling, kicking, or a combination in what is known as a "specific warm-down" (warming down from swimming by swimming very slowly), a "swim-down," "cool-down," "loosen-down," or just "easy." This mild exercising promotes circulation and removal of the fatigue products accumulated during the main part of your swimming workout. Some swimmers also like to do a "general warm-down" by repeating some or all of their stretching and flexibility exercises after they get out of the pool.

Note that whether or not a warm-down is written into the sample workouts in this book, you are advised to complete at least some type of specific warm-down procedure after your swimming workout. If the sample workouts don't have a listed warm-down, add several lengths on to the end of the workout as a very slow warm-down, or use the last few lengths of the written workout as the warm-down period before you get out of the pool.

Variety

The opportunities for variety in fitness swimming are limitless, and as such this area can provide a whole lifetime of active enjoyment. Despite initial enthusiasm, many people who start fitness programs eventually quit or continue in a very haphazard manner. It's easy to become bored if you don't know how to put variety into your workouts. Follow this advice and you'll never have to dread doing the same old thing over and over again. The following list is just a starting point of ideas for varying your swimming workouts:

• Mix it up—never do the same workout twice in a row or even more than once a month.

• Use different strokes for different parts of your workout.

• Swim a certain number of laps, or swim for a certain time period and don't even count laps!

• If the facility permits, swim over the short course (25 yards) at times and over the long course (50 meters) at other times.

• If the lanes are out, swim cross-pool or swim in the diving area.

• Occasionally skip a day, and sometimes do two workouts in one day.

• Try an early morning swim (this will wake you up), or swim late in the evening—under the stars is nice.

• Do some pulling, kicking, and swimming as part of your workout, and occasionally do a whole workout of just pulling, just kicking, or just swimming.

• Use a pull buoy to practice your hand action (with or without hand paddles). Use a kickboard to practice your kicks (with or without fins). Or kick without a kickboard.

• Use a pace clock to push hard. Or don't even think about your speed or times.

• Run on the pool bottom in shallow water. Or run in deep water, supported in a buoyant vest.

• Do some long swims in open water if you're near a beach. (Be sure to follow sensible safety precautions.)

• Take a break from swimming and do some other physical activity. Or do nothing at all.

Remember, a principal psychological benefit of exercise is diversity in your life, a pleasant change of pace in your daily routine. Don't grind out the same old swim every day.

The following "exercise prescription" summarizes some of the elements essential in planning your fitness-swimming program:

Type of exercise: fitness swimming.

Frequency: three or four times a week.

Intensity: target heart rate in the range of 100 to 160 beats per minute, adjusted according to age, swimming skill, and standard formula.

Duration: 30-minute workouts, after progressive buildup to this level.

Pattern: swim laps or swim for a time period, mostly with continuous swims. Alternate swimming and resting, however, when you first start fitness swimming (see Starter Workouts in Chapter 5).

Variety: deliberate and continual variations in distances, strokes, use of equipment, and the distribution of pulling, kicking, and swimming components.

Lifetime commitment: long-term involvement with aerobic exercise.

THREE

Standard Equipment

PERSONAL ITEMS PROVIDE comfort during fitness swimming, and exercise devices add challenge and variety to your training program. Besides swimsuit and goggles, there are four pieces of standard equipment that you should use occasionally in your fitness-swimming workouts: pull buoys, kickboards, hand paddles, and fins. If these devices are not supplied by the facility where you swim, you can purchase them yourself. Use these pieces of standard equipment to create variety in your exercise program. Be careful not to become overly dependent on any of these devices, especially the fins or pull buoy. More equipment items will be included later in the book for even more variations in your workouts.

SWIMSUIT. You can purchase an appropriate swimsuit at most sporting goods or department stores. Nylon suits dry out fastest between uses. Women will probably be more comfortable in one-piece suits, although two-piece suits can be worn. Men will probably be more comfortable in brief-style suits, although boxer trunks can be worn. After swimming, shower in your suit to rinse out the pool chemicals after you swim.

GOGGLES. A standard pair of goggles consists of two plastic lenses with soft rims around the inside edges, an elastic strap, and an adjustable nosepiece. Goggles permit you to see clearly underwater and keep the pool chemicals off your eyes. They come in a wide range of colors and shapes, and if you normally wear glasses, you can purchase goggles with your own prescription lenses in them. Write your name on the strap of the goggles in ballpoint ink in case you lose them. Keep spare parts from old goggles to make minor repairs.

It will take you a workout or two to get your goggles adjusted just right, with

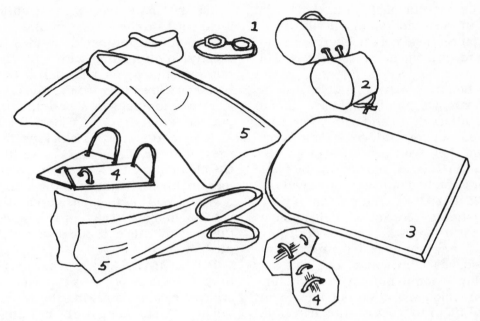

Equipment. Goggles (1), pull buoys, to keep your legs up while you work on your arm pulls (2), a kickboard, to keep your upper body buoyant while you practice kicks (3), hand paddles, which come in different styles (4), and fins or flippers, large or small (5).

the proper strap tension and nosepiece width. Wear the strap up a little high on the back of your head to create a good pull back into your eye sockets.

Just before you swim, you'll need to take preventive measures to keep your goggles from fogging up. Spit into them and rub the saliva around the insides of the lenses, then rinse them out and dump the contents into the pool gutter or drain. Shake out any extra drops of water, and you'll be ready to swim.

PULL BUOYS. Pull buoys consist of two buoyant foam cylinders bound together by an adjustable rope or molded together into one piece. They are used to practice the hand and arm movements of the various strokes. To use, hold the device lengthwise above the knees and work on your arm pull. Do not kick.

KICKBOARDS. Kickboards are flat, floating boards used to practice the kicking movements of the various strokes. They're made of a buoyant material and are available in different thicknesses, shapes, sizes, and colors.

To kick on your front, hold the board along its sides about one-third to two-thirds of the way up from the base end, keeping your thumbs on top and your fingers underneath. Keep your elbows straight and your shoulders at the surface of the water. The board should ride nearly flat on the surface of the water when you kick.

If you hold the top edge and get up on top of the kickboard too much, you'll weaken the kick by dropping the feet too low, and you may experience some lower back pain due to excessive arching.

To kick on your back, hold the board over your chest and stomach with your hands on each side of the board, or hold the board with one hand off to the side of your body.

You should occasionally kick without a kickboard. On your front, kick as usual with your face down and with your arms stretched out forward, breathing every now and then with a short arm stroke. On your back, keep your hands by your sides or stretched out over your head.

HAND PADDLES. Hand paddles have flat, plastic surfaces and are held against the hands by adjustable straps of rubber tubing. They are available in different sizes, shapes, and colors and add another dimension to pulling (using hands and arms alone). You do not kick—you just use them to work on the arm pull. Hand paddles will make you work a little harder and swim a little faster, and they will let you know if you're making any major mistakes in your stroke technique. Most often, hand paddles are used along with a pull buoy. For safety reasons, be careful not to hit any other swimmers with the paddles.

Hand paddles provide a good comparison with the normal hand position used in the various strokes and with the normal water pressure perceived through the hand. Two other interesting comparisons are to pull with the hands clenched ("fist swimming") and to pull while holding a tennis ball in each hand.

FINS. Fins, or flippers, make kicking possible and fun for many swimmers and give the legs a good workout. The large surface areas of the fins create greater force application, which leads to increased speed and efficiency in the water. Shoe-type fins are made of rubber, come in different brands and sizes, and enclose the entire foot.

Use the fins to kick with or without a kickboard, on the surface or underwater, and on your front, back, or sides. You'll mostly do fin kicking with a kickboard, but sometimes you will kick without a board or will swim with the fins on. Fins work well for kicks in which the toes are pointed, such as the fly kick, the back kick, and the crawl kick. Fins do not work well for the breast stroke kick or the elementary back kick, in which the toes are hooked up toward the shin.

When wearing fins, ease up a little on your push-offs after you turn, since the fins tend to "stick" to the pool wall if you push off hard.

POOL MARKINGS. *Surface lane lines* are made of colored plastic floats on a wire cable, breaking the water turbulence and dividing the swimming pool into lanes. The float colors are mixed in the center span and are solid for the last 15 feet at each end. Never sit on, hang on, or lift up the surface lane lines, since they can be stretched or broken.

One swimmer can swim alone right in the middle of the surface lane lines. Two swimmers can use the same lane if each keeps to his or her own side of the lane (using half the lane). Three or more swimmers can use the same lane by "circling," going down one side of the lane and then back along the other side (usually counterclockwise). These swimmers must be spaced out within the lane at least 5 to 8 yards apart to reduce the chance of swimming into each other.

Back stroke flags are suspended across the pool 7 feet over the surface and 15 feet from the wall, enabling back stroke swimmers to anticipate their turns or finishes. Good swimmers can pass under the flags and then count the number of strokes needed to get to a hand touch on the wall, while less skilled

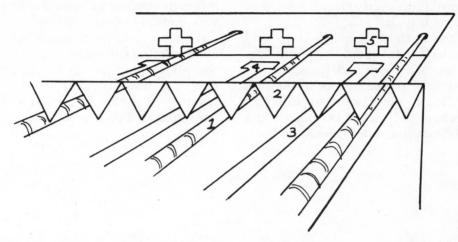

Standard Pool Markings. Surface lane lines (1), back stroke flags overhead (2), bottom lane line down the middle of each lane (3), with a T at each end (4), and targets on the pool wall (5).

swimmers need to look for the wall over one shoulder once or twice prior to the hand touch.

Bottom lane lines (usually black) run along the pool bottom in the exact middle between the surface lane lines, ending in a T shape 5 feet from the wall. They enable you to swim straight, to anticipate your turn or finish, and to maintain a traffic pattern within your lane.

A cross-shaped *target* (also usually black) is centered on the pool wall in each lane, another marking to help you to anticipate your turn or finish.

SPECIAL-EQUIPMENT WORKOUT. The following workout is a good summary of how to use the standard equipment presented in this chapter. Most fitness swimmers should be able to do these procedures, even if just for one length each. Try it—you may not like every component, but this workout (22 lengths total) shows you many different ways of using the equipment. *P* means pulling, and *K* means kicking.

With a pull buoy, 6 lengths, arms alone:

    crawl P
    back P
    breast P
    elementary back P
    crawl P, right arm only
    crawl P, left arm only

With a kickboard, 4 lengths, legs alone:

    crawl K
    back K
    breast K
    elementary back K

With a pull buoy and hand paddles, 4 lengths, arms alone:

    crawl P
    back P
    breast P
    elementary back P

With a kickboard and fins, 8 lengths, legs alone:

    crawl K
    back K
    fly K

crawl K on right side
crawl K on left side
crawl K, right leg only
crawl K, left leg only
crawl K without a kickboard

The basic principle in this workout is variety. Mix it up; always do different things when you swim. Do not do the same workout time after time. Use 3 or 4 different strokes in your workouts, and you can break any stroke down into arms alone and then legs alone, as well as swimming the entire stroke. Purchase the above four pieces of equipment if they are not provided by the facility where you swim. Work on both your strengths and your weaknesses.

FOUR

Breathing Exercises

AN AEROBIC EXERCISE (an exercise that uses oxygen) like swimming depends completely on continual air exchange—inhalation and exhalation—especially during heavy exertion. You will become uncomfortable or extremely fatigued if you gasp for air, inhale water, or hold your breath while you swim. People who don't learn to breathe easily in the pool usually tend to avoid fitness swimming. Work on your breathing patterns in various strokes so that you can sustain your fitness swimming long enough to benefit from it. Steady, rhythmic breathing is the key, and with practice you'll soon feel comfortable breathing as you swim.

The procedures in this chapter form a rough progression for learning alternate-side breathing in crawl stroke and should help with your breathing in the other strokes, too.

You can practice breathing as part of your fitness-swimming workouts, or in special sessions devoted just to breathing patterns. When you're starting your exercise program, work on these procedures frequently until you reach the goal of full air exchange during the various swimming strokes and skills.

Concentrate on breathing in through your mouth above the water and out slowly through your nose down into the water. (When you're working hard, some air will also be exhaled through your mouth without your having to think about it.) This sets up a rhythmic pattern and prevents water from rushing up into your nose.

Holding your breath while you swim would lead to oxygen debt (not enough oxygen), which would wipe you out physically and greatly reduce the distances you can swim. Trying to both exhale and then inhale as you turn or lift your head above the water can also lead to oxygen debt, since at that point in your stroke there is not enough time to perform both actions. When you turn or lift your head, all you should have to do is breathe in. When your face is down, exhale, especially through your nose. Whenever your face is down, keep your eyes focused on the bottom of the pool about 2 to 4 feet in front of you.

In the crawl, good swimmers do not swim flat on the surface of the water. They roll from side to side, as much as 45 to 50 degrees each way. Try to add more momentum and freedom of motion to your crawl by using more shoulder and body roll coordinated with your breathing. This adds power to your underwater pulls and makes the recovery of your arms easier.

The neck itself doesn't turn much (maybe not at all) when you breathe in crawl, as the hands, arms, shoulders, neck, and head all work together to position your open mouth to breathe in a small pocket of air formed by the side of your face, your forward momentum through the water, and your shoulder roll.

The ability to breathe to both sides in crawl (alternate-side breathing) provides fitness swimmers with several benefits:

• It will make your stroke more equal on both sides. If you only breathe to one side, your arm stroke on that side tends to be stronger and more propulsive.

• It reduces tension. There is often tension in the shoulder of the arm on the nonbreathing side, especially during the recovery (the return of the arm over the surface), because it usually rides a little lower in the water than the other shoulder. Alternate-side breathing reduces this tension, making the shoulder less susceptible to pain or injury.

• It enables you to breathe whenever you want to whichever side you want. You maintain a level of comfort and the ability to be "in charge" of your own breathing rather than being controlled by a desperate need for air.

BOBBING. Bobbing is the most basic breathing exercise in the water. While standing on the pool bottom in shoulder-deep water, bend your knees until your head is completely submerged. Then stand up again just enough that your mouth is above the water surface. Look forward and coordinate these down-and-up movements with a continuous in-the-mouth and out-the-nose breathing pattern. Exhale slowly through your nose both on the way down and on the way up through the water. In time, you will become accustomed to breathing with water running down over your hair, eyes, nose, and mouth as your head comes up above the water surface. Keep your head still: don't shake it around or you'll lose the bobbing rhythm.

Once you're comfortable in shoulder-deep water, you can practice in deeper water (6 to 8 feet). Push down with your arms and legs to lift yourself up a little above the water surface. Descend vertically underwater with your legs together and your arms by your sides. Push off the pool bottom to return to the surface, just high enough to breathe in through your mouth before going under again. Remember to exhale through your nose all the way down and back up through the water. *Travel bobbing* is a variation in which you lean forward slightly during each push from the pool bottom, ascending to the surface each time at a slight angle.

If the deep water in your pool is very deep, you can do *ladder bobbing* by holding on to the rungs or sides of a pool

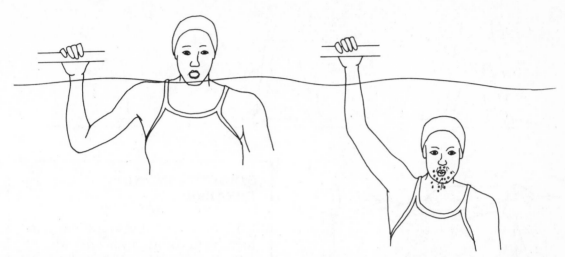

Bobbing: Breathe in through your mouth. Submerge and exhale through your nose. Keep exhaling as you return to the surface. Stay slow and steady, repeating these down-and-up movements over and over again. Do not shake your head.

ladder. Let yourself down underwater to full extension, then pull yourself back up, breathing as described above.

Consider using bobbing for a minute or two as a relaxing way of finishing a workout, simply bobbing until your breathing returns to a more normal state. This is an excellent method of concluding a workout.

STANDING AND SIDE BREATHING. Side breathing—one step beyond bobbing—can be learned by standing on the bottom and holding the pool gutter. Bend forward to a swimming-like position and breathe to both the right side and the left side. Then alternate sides: right, left, right, left. You'll need to bend your elbows very slightly and roll your shoulders to reach a breathing position while standing. A common mistake is to lift the head and look forward before turning the head to the side. Keep the water surface at or slightly above your hairline, and breathe only to the side.

Body roll is important: you should be flat only when your face is down in the water. Keep your rhythm slow and steady—remember, you're in charge.

The following are some variations of this breathing exercise beyond just standing:

• While still holding the gutter with your hands, get your feet off the pool bottom with a slow, easy flutter kick (crawl kick) to simulate a swimming position even more.

• Add some forward momentum by flutter-kicking with a kickboard while doing the breathing drills to the right, left, and alternate sides.

• If you don't have a strong kick, use fins along with the kickboard to create movement through the water.

STANDING, STROKING, AND SIDE BREATHING. Breathing patterns for stroking can be learned while standing in water that is waist-deep to chest-deep. Bend forward to simulate swimming the

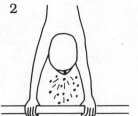

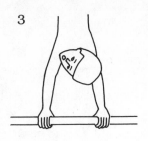

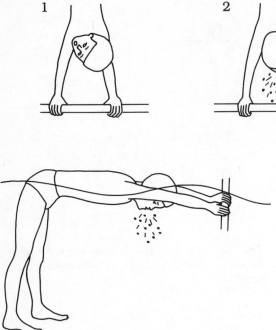

STANDING AND SIDE
BREATHING

1. Turn your face to the side and
breathe in through your mouth.
2. Turn your face down and
exhale through your nose.
3. Turn your face to the side and
breathe in through your mouth
again. Stay slow and steady,
repeating the total breathing cycle
over and over again.

crawl, keeping your feet on the pool bottom. Brace yourself with your hands holding the pool gutter and bend your knees slightly. If you're breathing to the right, put your left leg forward a little; if to the left, advance your right leg. If you're alternating breathing sides, keep your feet even.

When you start to stroke, move your hands slowly enough that you don't pull yourself out of your braced, stationary position. Begin right-sided breathing when the right hand and arm reach the level of the right shoulder in the underwater pull. Breathing to that side is completed as the underwater pull is finished. Then turn your face back down as the hand and arm move over the surface into

the recovery. Left-sided breathing is done in a similar fashion to the left side. If you wait until your hand is back by your hip or leg before turning to breathe, you are breathing too late. You must start to breathe sooner.

If your head is turning to the side to breathe as your arm is starting to recover over the water, you will have created two opposing motions, which will disrupt your stroking rhythm. Also, the recovering arm often carries some water on it which can be thrown into your face. This distracts beginners and makes them uncomfortable in their initial breathing attempts.

Breathe early, as the hand and arm start to pull back underwater; then all of the movements of the hand, arm, shoulders, head, and neck will begin to fit together smoothly in a coordinated breathing pattern. Shoulder roll or body roll is an important component in successful breathing.

Practicing the various breathing patterns (right side, left side, alternate sides) in a standing position is an extremely important step for beginning fitness swimmers who experience breathing difficulties or for those who are learning new patterns. In time, that same relaxed feeling you can get as you breathe while standing, stroking, and side breathing can transfer into your stroke as you move through the water. It can feel the same—really!

With slight modification, this procedure will work well for learning to breathe in the butterfly and breast strokes, too. You can also use this exercise as a quick review if you have occasional problems with your breathing in any of the face-down strokes.

CRAWL STROKE BREATHING.

There are three basic breathing patterns for the crawl, plus two combination patterns:

Right side only. Breathe during every stroke to the right as you swim. A few swimmers can breathe every other stroke to the right side, but most need the oxygen delivered with breathing every stroke to one side.

Left side only. Breathe during every stroke to the left as you swim. Again, a few swimmers may breathe every other stroke to the left side.

Basic alternate-side breathing (one right and one left). Breathe to alternate sides during every third arm stroke. You cannot turn your head fast enough to breathe during every single arm stroke to alternate sides. You must skip an arm stroke to breathe every third stroke. Keep exhaling slowly through your nose while your face is down. A large number of fitness swimmers like this pattern once they break away from one-sided swimming.

Alternate-side breathing (two right and two left). Breathe to the right side two times consecutively, skip an arm stroke, breathe to the left side two times consecutively, skip an arm stroke, and repeat this pattern. Slow down—think it through. Concentrate on exhaling when your face is down. This pattern simply combines the three previous patterns into a new way of breathing. Some swimmers like this alternate-side pattern because they don't have to turn the head back and forth as frequently.

Alternate-side breathing (four or more right and four or more left). Breathe right four or more times consecutively, skip an arm stroke, breathe left four or more times consecutively, skip an arm stroke, and repeat. In this pattern you breathe longer to one side before switching to the other side.

Some swimmers alternate by lengths, breathing to the right side on the way down the pool and to the left on the way back, and some alternate lengths of basic alternate-side breathing with lengths of single-side breathing.

If you have trouble with the last two breathing patterns, try them while doing the standing, stroking, and side-breathing drill. You can pick them up more easily in a stationary position than while actually swimming.

There are other ways to practice all five breathing patterns for the crawl. Use

STANDING, STROKING, AND SIDE BREATHING

1. Exhale through your nose with your face down.
2. Start your right arm pull; turn your head to the side as your arm approaches shoulder level in the pull. Keep exhaling through the nose.
3. With your head turned to the side (not lifted up), breathe in through your mouth.
4. Finish breathing in through your mouth as your arm is pulled all the way back.
5. Turn your face down and exhale through your nose, continuing to exhale as your hand and arm move over the surface in the recovery.
6. Keep exhaling slowly through your nose. Stroke once with your left arm, then repeat the total breathing cycle over and over again.

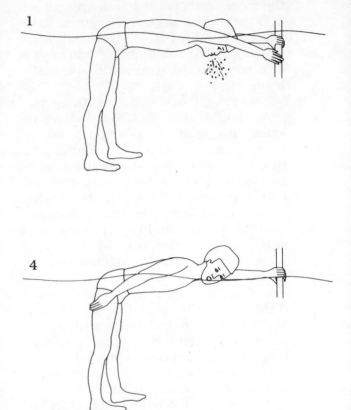

the following methods as you learn to breathe or add them to your workouts for more variety:

• *Swim bubble.* For a beginning fitness swimmer who has great difficulty learning to breathe, a child's swim bubble can permit him or her to move and try the breathing without sinking. Sometimes, two bubbles (a double bubble) are needed to provide enough security to permit the swimmer to calm down and learn how to breathe comfortably. For a few swimmers, this can be a slow process. As they're more successful, they can gradually be weaned away from the flotation device. This has been a very helpful step with scared or very inexperienced beginners. The bubble works just like training wheels on a bicycle.

• *Pull buoy.* Hold a pull buoy above your knees and between your legs lengthwise. Don't kick; just concentrate on learning the various breathing patterns with the slight buoyant assist of the device.

• *One-arm swimming.* This may be

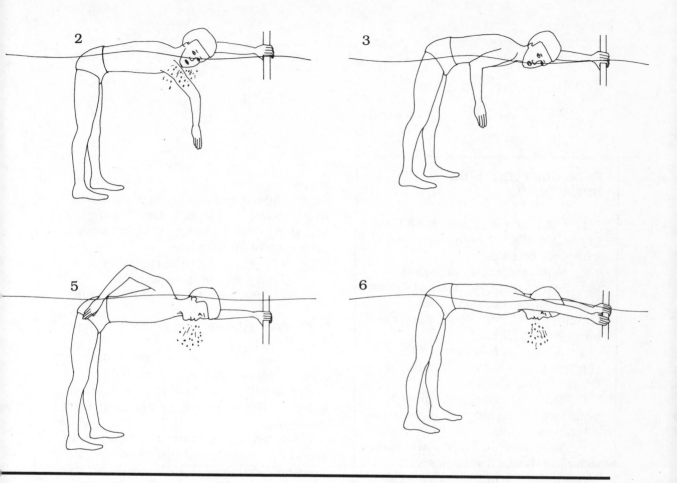

done with or without a pull buoy. To use your right arm, hold your left hand and arm straight out in front of your left shoulder. You'll instinctively want to move this arm, but you must keep it still and steady. Stroke only with your right hand and arm, and breathe only to the right side. To use your left arm, keep your right arm out straight, stroke only with your left arm, and breathe only to the left. This drill usually alternates right-arm-only lengths with left-arm-only lengths. It strengthens both the arm pull and the side-breathing patterns.

• *Fins.* Swim crawl with fins on. The fins give you a big boost in power, which can help you learn new ways of breathing.

• *Weak side first.* To develop your weaker side, breathe to that side as you come out of every turn and push-off for one or two arm strokes before continuing with the breathing pattern you have chosen for the rest of the length.

SPECIAL BREATHING WORKOUT. The following workout is a good sum-

1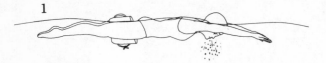

2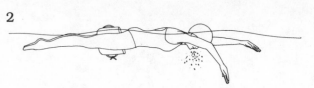

PULL BUOY AND SIDE BREATHING

1. Hold the pull buoy above your knees. Exhale through your nose with your face down.

2. Begin your right arm pull.

3. Start turning your head to the side as your arm approaches shoulder level in the pull. Keep exhaling through your nose.

4. With your head turned to the side (not lifted up), breathe in through your mouth.

5. Finish breathing in through your mouth as your arm is pulled all the way back.

6. Turn your face down and keep exhaling through your nose, as your right arm recovers and as your left arm pull begins.

7. Keep exhaling slowly through your nose.

8. Your left arm begins its recovery, then repeat the total breathing cycle over and over again.

mary requiring you to use all of the breathing patterns for crawl presented in this chapter. Repeat the following breathing pattern twice, all crawl stroke, for a total of 20 lengths:

> 2 lengths—breathe right side
> 2 lengths—breathe left side
> 2 lengths—alternate sides (1 right, 1 left)
> 2 lengths—alternate sides (2 right, 2 left)
> 2 lengths—alternate sides (4 or more right, 4 or more left)

For variety, continue to use different crawl stroke breathing patterns in your workouts.

Work on both your strengths and weaknesses in breathing patterns. Remember your goal of full, steady air exchange as you swim. Develop your breathing in the other strokes, too.

OTHER STROKES

All of the breathing exercises in this

5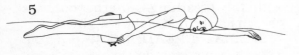

6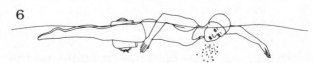

3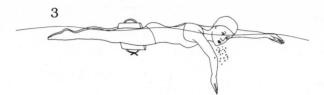

4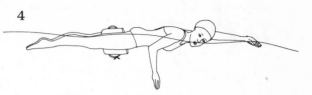

chapter can be modified a little to contribute to success in breathing in the other strokes as well. As you read the descriptions below, look at the stroke illustrations in Chapter 8 to help you to visualize the breathing patterns in these other strokes.

Your goal is to breathe fully and comfortably without even thinking about it while you swim.

BREAST STROKE. In the breast stroke, you'll breathe to the front (looking forward) during each arm stroke. This seems to fit the rhythm of this stroke best. When the arms sweep in under your shoulders, your upper body and head will rise up in the water. This is the most natural time to breathe in this stroke. Breast stroke has the most up-and-down movement of all the strokes. Your breathing must be coordinated with the rising up, falling forward, stretching out, and gliding parts of the stroke.

BACK STROKES. In the back stroke and elementary back stroke, since your face is up as you swim, there is no one right time to breathe, and you can breathe whenever you want. It is important, however, to breathe on a regular cycle so that you don't hold your breath for extended periods of time. Most swimmers inhale during the arm recovery and exhale during the underwater pull.

BUTTERFLY STROKE. In the butterfly stroke, you'll breathe to the front as hands and arms reach the level of the shoulders in the underwater pull. The breathing will be done as your hands and arms finish the pull and swing out and over into the recovery. Breathing every second stroke seems best for this stroke; keep your face down on the alternate strokes. Usually, you'll look forward (put your chin on the surface of the water) as you breathe. A very small number of swimmers are successful at breathing to the side in this stroke.

7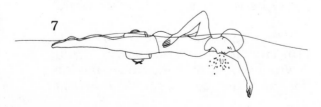

8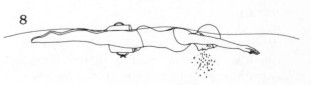

SHELBYVILLE-SHELBY COUNTY
PUBLIC LIBRARY

FIVE

Lap-Swimming Workouts

A PRINCIPAL METHOD of fitness-swimming training is to swim a predetermined distance (20 lengths, 50 lengths, or whatever) continuously for your entire exercise period. Once you get established, you will likely swim different distances on different days. Since nothing is more important than your consistent participation over a long period of time, this chapter provides plenty of lap-swimming workouts to complete in the pool.

It's more fun to do these workouts than to read about them. Study this chapter enough to understand the introductory concepts and then to see how the sets of each workout fit together. There are lap workouts ranging from starter workouts for beginners to the highest-range workouts for top fitness swimmers. In time, you will become skilled at creating your own personalized workouts, exploring the tremendous variety that makes fitness swimming interesting as a lifetime activity.

In these lap-swimming workouts, the variable is distance, as measured by the number of lengths that you swim:

> 1 length = down the pool = 25 yards
> 1 lap = 2 lengths = down and back = 50 yards = 1 round trip

Most swimmers keep track of their lengths in their mind as they swim, usually with an ascending count by ones. Some swimmers count laps instead of lengths. You can construct a lap counter, using beads or washers on a thin dowel, to keep track of your count. Some people move coins on the side of the pool. Clicking types of adding devices are useful, too.

If there are some empty lanes near your lane, it's fun to do "snakes," going down one lane, ducking under the lane line, and then coming back in another lane. This pattern also helps with counting lengths. For example, if you go over four lanes and then back four lanes, you know you've done 8 lengths without really having to think about your count. Variations include snakes by twos (going down and back in the same lane, then moving to the next lane) and snakes by a variable number (for example, 8 lengths in lane one, 6 lengths in lane two, 4 lengths in lane three, 2 lengths in lane four). If lanes are crowded, you could go down in one lane and then back in the next lane, circling counterclockwise in just two lanes.

FINDING YOUR STARTING POINT. This section will be most helpful to beginning fitness swimmers who lack experience in this form of exercise. If you've been swimming for fitness for a while, you'll already know where you fit into these sample workouts, and you'll be able to relate the distances you can swim to the amount of time you'll need to finish the workouts.

Beginners can test themselves by seeing how far they can swim at one time without stopping and without pushing excessively. Roughly, this is your starting point in this program. Begin somewhere around this starting point to build yourself up slowly (see next section) over a period of two to eight weeks of fitness swimming.

Ultimately, your daily program will vary in distance from day to day (see Random-Distance Programs). Having done the buildup, you can swim just about any distance you choose on any day.

PROGRESSIVE BUILDUPS. If you're at a relatively low starting point, you'll need to start your fitness-swimming workouts slowly, carefully, and progres-

sively. If you're a true beginner in this activity, you could simply begin with the first starter lap-swimming workout given below and build up through all twenty workouts listed. This approach should develop your confidence and endurance to go beyond this range.

The following types of buildups have worked well in our fitness-swimming courses over the years. A starting point of 20 lengths is assumed, but you can project the following progressive patterns down to lower starting points if needed for a longer buildup.

- Sixteen days:
  20–20–24
  28–28–32
  36–36–40
  44–44–48
  52–52–60
  test at 70 (1 mile).
- Sixteen days:
  20–24–24
  28–32–32
  36–40–40
  44–48–48
  52–56–56
  test at 70.
- Twelve days:
  20–24–28–32–36
  40–44–48–52–56
  60–test at 70.

Remember, these are just examples. Be sure to follow the basic principle of building yourself up gradually from one workout to the next in terms of your distances and effort.

RANDOM-DISTANCE PROGRAMS. In time you'll reach the point where you can handle just about any distance in your workouts. You'll probably vary your distance from day to day, sometimes doing a longer workout and other times a little shorter. How much time you have available to swim on a certain day will be a factor in determining the distance of your workout.

The following types of random patterns have worked well in our fitness-swimming courses over the years. A minimum of 40 lengths is assumed, but you can project the random patterns down lower if needed.

- Thirteen days:
  40–50–46–54–42–58–44–52–48–56–60–70–test at 100.
- Fourteen days:
  40–50–60–70–50–60–40–60–50–70–60–50–40–test at 100.

Remember, again these are just examples. Your workouts will likely vary from 15 to 45 minutes, with an average duration of 30 minutes of exercise. Mixing up your distances randomly from one workout to the next will help you create variety in your training program.

SAMPLE WORKOUTS. The sample workouts in this book are good as written but should not be regarded as absolutes. You may modify them or combine parts of several different workouts to construct a workout that meets your own special needs and interests on any given day.

Workouts are made up of sets. Which are line items or definite units that develop each part of the workout. Subsets are brief explanations of the way in which the set is to be completed. For example, one line of a longer workout might be summarized "10 lengths breast stroke." Here, ten lengths is the set and breast stroke is the subset. A set may be a number of lengths all of the same stroke, or a number of lengths of different strokes. Remember to swim it without stopping to rest. You may not be able to do so right away, but that's your goal: swim each set without stopping. One set in a long workout, for example, may read, "10 lengths breast," and the next set may read, "6 lengths crawl." Swim the 10 lengths of breast stroke without a break, then stop to catch your breath before swimming the 6 lengths of crawl at least as a beginning fitness swimmer. Any number in the subsets also refer to lengths.

A more complicated set may read,

12 lengths:
   2 crawl
+ 4 breast
+ 2 crawl
+ 4 elementary back

Swim the set of 12 lengths without stopping between the subsets. That is, go straight from the 2 lengths of crawl to the 4 lengths of breast stroke, and so forth. The indents and the plus signs (+) are our signal that the subsets together equal one continuous 12-length swim, with the strokes changing as specified.

Ultimately you will probably want to tie all the sets of an entire workout together into one continuous swim. But you may want or need to rest a minute or two between workout sets, especially as you are building yourself up in fitness swimming.

Remember to check your heart rate from time to time to make sure you're in a range that is safe but will also maximize your training benefits.

If the particular way listed to complete a set or subset is not to your liking or ability, change it—substitute something else. If you repeat a workout sometime in the future, you may want to do each set or subset slightly differently. As you gain experience, construct your own workouts by creating new combinations and variations of things to do.

TERMS. Although most subset notations are self-explanatory, some common symbols and abbreviations used in the sample workouts throughout this book are explained here.

Easy. Another term for warm-up or warm-down; also a slower swim between faster swims in the middle of a workout.

Fitness medley (FM). Doing the four basic fitness strokes in this order: crawl, back, breast, elementary back; often done by single lengths, but could be by twos, threes, or any number, or numbers of lengths could vary for each stroke.

Fly. Butterfly.

K. Kicking—using just the legs on your front, back, or side, with or without a kickboard, and with or without fins.

Mixer. A long swim changing strokes frequently but in random patterns; might include some pulling, kicking, and swimming plus other variations.

On your back. Pulling, kicking, or swimming the back stroke or the elementary back stroke; you have some choice with this subset.

P. Pulling—using just the arms; with a pull buoy but no kicking; with or without hand paddles; usually with crawl but can be done with the other strokes, too.

R–L. One-arm swimming usually using the right arm only (R) down the pool and the left arm only (L) back; usually with crawl but can be done with the other strokes, too. Also refers to breathing to the right side and then to the left side in a repeating pattern while swimming the crawl, such as 1 length breathing to the right alternated with 1 length breathing to the left. May also refer to kicking on the right side and then on the left in a repeating pattern for crawl (or fly) kicks, such as 1 length kicking on the right side followed by 1 length kicking on the left.

Reverse FM. A fitness medley taking the fitness strokes in reverse order: elementary back, breast, back, crawl.

S. Swimming the whole stroke, with pulling and kicking combined; if not specified otherwise, S is always intended in the subset.

Sequences. Can be developed for different lengths of a set; for example, "1 P + 1 K + 1 jog + 1 K + 1 S" means pull a length, kick a length, water jog a length, kick a length, and swim a length, in that order and preferably continuously.

Stroke. Any stroke except the crawl: back, breast, elementary back, or butterfly.

Stroke mixer. A long swim using several strokes but not including the crawl, changing strokes often but in no particular order.

Water jogging. Running on the pool bottom in shallow water.

Starter Lap-Swimming Workouts

The following workouts of 10 lengths or fewer are for beginning fitness swim-mers. It is assumed that you will do a lot of swimming and resting as you build your way up to continuous workouts.

WORKOUT 1	Dates Completed		
1 length on your front			
1 length on your back			
2 total			

WORKOUT 2	Dates Completed		
1 length P			
1 length K			
2 total			

WORKOUT 3	Dates Completed		
Swim continuously:			
1 length crawl			
1 length breast			
2 total			

WORKOUT 4	Dates Completed		
2 lengths crawl continuous			
2 total			

WORKOUT 5	Dates Completed		
2 lengths breast			
2 lengths elementary back			
4 total			

WORKOUT 6	Dates Completed		
Fitness medley (FM):			
1 length crawl			
1 length back			
1 length breast			
1 length elementary back			
4 total			

WORKOUT 7	Dates Completed		
Swim continuously, all with fins:			
1 length K			
+ 1 length crawl			
+ 1 length K			
+ 1 length crawl			
4 total			

WORKOUT 8	Dates Completed		
4 lengths crawl continuous			
4 total			

WORKOUT 9	Dates Completed		
2 lengths P			
2 lengths K with fins			
2 lengths crawl			
6 total			

WORKOUT 10	Dates Completed		
1 length crawl			
1 length on your back			
1 length breast			
1 length crawl			
1 length on your back			
1 length breast			
6 total			

WORKOUT 11	Dates Completed		
1 length K			
2 lengths crawl			
2 lengths breast			
1 length K			
6 total			

WORKOUT 12	Dates Completed		
6 lengths crawl continuous			
6 total			

WORKOUT 13	Dates Completed		
4 lengths:			
2 P			
+ 2 K			
4 lengths:			
2 breast			
+ 2 elementary back			
8 total			

WORKOUT 14	Dates Completed		
2 lengths breast			
4 lengths crawl			
2 lengths on your back			
8 total			

WORKOUT 15	Dates Completed		
FM:			
2 lengths crawl			
2 lengths back			
2 lengths breast			
2 lengths elementary back			
8 total			

WORKOUT 16	Dates Completed		
8 lengths crawl			
8 total			

WORKOUT 17	Dates Completed		
2 lengths P			
2 lengths K			
2 lengths P			
2 lengths K			
2 lengths P			
10 total			

WORKOUT 18	Dates Completed		
4 lengths crawl			
3 lengths back			
2 lengths breast			
1 length elementary back			
10 total			

WORKOUT 19	Dates Completed		
5 lengths any one stroke			
5 lengths something completely different			
10 total			

WORKOUT 20	Dates Completed		
10 lengths crawl			
10 total			

Low-Range Lap-Swimming Workouts

These workouts of 10 to 30 lengths should take a rough minimum of 5 to 15 minutes for the fastest fitness swimmers, and longer for most others. You should gradually be doing more continuous swimming and less resting as you make your way through these workouts.

WORKOUT 21	Dates Completed		
2 lengths K			
6 lengths any one stroke			
2 lengths water jogging			
10 total			

WORKOUT 22	Dates Completed		
9 lengths:			
1 P			
+ 1 K			
+ 1 S			
(x3)			
1 length easy			
10 total			

WORKOUT 23	Dates Completed		
2 lengths on your back			
4 lengths breast			
6 lengths:			
1 R			
+1 L			
+1 regular crawl			
(x2)			
12 total			

WORKOUT 24	Dates Completed		
3 lengths P crawl with hand paddles			
3 lengths fin K crawl			
3 lengths crawl			
3 lengths elementary back			
12 total			

WORKOUT 25	Dates Completed		
2 lengths:			
1 K			
+ 1 water jogging			
6 lengths crawl			
4 lengths breast			
2 lengths easy			
14 total			

WORKOUT 26	Dates Completed		
4 lengths:			
1 K			
+ 1 P			
(x2)			
8 lengths crawl			
2 lengths easy			
14 total			

WORKOUT 27

	Dates Completed		

1 length easy
5 lengths crawl
4 lengths back
3 lengths breast
2 lengths elementary back
1 length easy
_____
16 total

WORKOUT 28

	Dates Completed		

4 lengths crawl
4 lengths breast
4 lengths crawl
4 lengths on your back
_____
16 total

WORKOUT 29	Dates Completed		
3 lengths K			
6 lengths:			
2 back			
+ 2 breast			
+ 2 elementary back			
9 lengths crawl			
18 total			

WORKOUT 30	Dates Completed		
1 length K, no kickboard			
4 lengths crawl			
8 lengths:			
2 crawl			
+ 1 water jogging			
+ 2 breast			
+ 1 water jogging			
+ 2 elementary back			
4 lengths crawl			
1 length K, no kickboard			
18 total			

WORKOUT 31	Dates Completed		
2 lengths K			
4 lengths breast			
8 lengths crawl			
4 lengths back or elementary back			
2 lengths K			
20 total			

WORKOUT 32	Dates Completed		
20 lengths stroke mixer, no crawl			
20 total			

WORKOUT 33	Dates Completed		
1 length easy			
2 lengths back			
4 lengths crawl			
8 lengths breast			
4 lengths crawl			
2 lengths elementary back			
1 length easy			
22 total			

WORKOUT 34	Dates Completed		
7 lengths P crawl			
7 lengths fin K			
7 lengths stroke mixer, no crawl			
1 length water jogging			
22 total			

WORKOUT 35

	Dates Completed		

4 lengths crawl
4 lengths breast
4 lengths back or elementary back
4 lengths crawl
4 lengths breast
4 lengths back or elementary back

24 total

WORKOUT 36

	Dates Completed		

 6 lengths breast or back
12 lengths crawl
 6 lengths:

    1½ elementary back
  + ½ water jogging
    (x3)

24 total

WORKOUT 37	Dates Completed		
10 lengths crawl			
8 lengths fin K on your back			
6 lengths breast			
2 lengths easy			
26 total			

WORKOUT 38	Dates Completed		
2 lengths easy			
4 lengths crawl			
8 lengths breast			
12 lengths:			
8 lengths crawl			
+ 4 lengths easy			
26 total			

WORKOUT 39	Dates Completed		
7 lengths breast			
14 lengths crawl			
7 lengths on your back			
28 total			

WORKOUT 40	Dates Completed		
7 completely different sets of 4 lengths each			
28 total			

WORKOUT 41	Dates Completed		
15 lengths crawl			
10 lengths strokes only			
5 lengths K			
30 total			

WORKOUT 42	Dates Completed		
6 lengths P crawl			
6 lengths fin K			
6 lengths P crawl with hand paddles			
6 lengths stroke mixer, no crawl			
6 lengths:			
½ K			
+ ½ water jogging			
(x6)			
30 total			

Mid-Range Lap-Swimming Workouts

These workouts of 30 to 50 lengths should take a rough minimum of 15 to 25 minutes for the fastest fitness swimmers, and longer for most others. You'll be using mostly continuous swimming with only occasional resting as you go through these workouts. This is the range in which a large number of fitness swimmers participate.

WORKOUT 43	Dates Completed		
6 lengths crawl			
4 lengths back			
6 lengths crawl			
4 lengths breast			
6 lengths crawl			
4 lengths elementary back			
30 total			

WORKOUT 44	Dates Completed		
20 lengths crawl			
10 lengths breast			
30 total			

WORKOUT 45	Dates Completed		
32 lengths P crawl			
32 total			

WORKOUT 46	Dates Completed		
4 lengths crawl			
8 lengths breast			
12 lengths crawl			
6 lengths:			
1 back			
+ 2 elementary back			
(x2)			
2 lengths crawl			
32 total			

WORKOUT 47	Dates Completed		
2 lengths elementary back			
12 lengths breast			
6 lengths K			
12 lengths back			
2 lengths water jogging			
34 total			

WORKOUT 48	Dates Completed		
8 lengths crawl			
8 lengths:			
1 elementary back			
+ 1 back			
(x4)			
8 lengths:			
1 fly K			
+ 1 breast			
(x4)			
8 lengths crawl			
2 lengths easy			
34 total			

WORKOUT 49	Dates Completed		
9 lengths P crawl			
9 lengths continuous, all fin K:			
3 lengths fly			
+ 3 lengths back			
+ 3 lengths crawl			
18 lengths mixer, all strokes			
36 total			

WORKOUT 50	Dates Completed		
24 lengths crawl			
12 lengths:			
1 back			
+ 2 breast			
+ 1 elementary back			
(x3)			
36 total			

WORKOUT 51	Dates Completed		
3 lengths easy			
10 lengths:			
1 K			
+ 1 stroke			
(x5)			
5 lengths crawl with flip turns (optional)			
20 lengths P crawl			
38 total			

WORKOUT 52	Dates Completed		
6 lengths easy			
15 lengths stroke mixer, no crawl			
10 lengths:			
1 K			
+ 1 S			
(x5)			
5 lengths crawl			
2 lengths easy			
38 total			

WORKOUT 53	Dates Completed		
10 lengths crawl			
2 lengths fly K			
4 lengths breast			
6 lengths back			
8 lengths breast			
10 lengths crawl			
40 total			

WORKOUT 54	Dates Completed		
40 lengths breast stroke only			
40 total			

WORKOUT 55	Dates Completed		
42 lengths:			
6 crawl + 1 breast			
+ 5 crawl + 2 breast			
+ 4 crawl + 3 breast			
+ 3 crawl + 4 breast			
+ 2 crawl + 5 breast			
+ 1 crawl + 6 breast			
42 total			

WORKOUT 56	Dates Completed		
6 lengths:			
1 fly K			
+ 1 stroke			
(x3)			
18 lengths crawl			
12 lengths breast			
6 lengths:			
1 water jogging			
+ 1 stroke			
(x3)			
42 total			

WORKOUT 57	Dates Completed		
16 lengths P crawl			
4 lengths fin K			
16 lengths:			
2 crawl			
+ 2 back			
+ 2 breast			
+ 2 elementary back			
(x2)			
4 lengths K			
4 lengths easy			
44 total			

WORKOUT 58	Dates Completed		
2 lengths easy			
4 lengths FM K, no fins, no kickboard			
8 lengths crawl			
12 lengths:			
2 back			
+ 2 breast			
(x3)			
16 lengths P crawl:			
1 R			
+ 1 L			
+ 2 regular crawl			
(x4)			
2 lengths easy			
44 total			

WORKOUT 59	Dates Completed		
4 lengths easy			
40 lengths stroke mixer			
2 lengths easy			
46 total			

WORKOUT 60	Dates Completed		
4 lengths easy P			
18 lengths crawl with slow pace			
2 lengths easy stroke			
18 lengths crawl with faster pace			
4 lengths easy K			
46 total			

WORKOUT 61

	Dates Completed	

4 lengths breast
2 lengths P crawl R-L
2 lengths try crawl with flip turn
4 lengths:
     1 back
   + 1 elementary back
    (x2)
2 lengths P crawl R-L
2 lengths try crawl with flip turn

16 lengths
(x3)

48 total

WORKOUT 62

	Dates Completed	

12 lengths P crawl with hand paddles
 4 lengths fly K
12 lengths:
    1 back
   + 1 breast
   + 2 elementary back
    (x3)
 4 lengths back K
12 lengths crawl
 4 lengths crawl K

48 total

WORKOUT 63 | Dates Completed

10 lengths crawl:
   1 breathe R
 + 1 breathe L
   (x5)
10 lengths crawl breathe R only
10 lengths crawl breathe L only
10 lengths crawl breathe to alternate sides
10 lengths crawl:
   1 breathe R
 + 1 breathe L
   (x5)

50 total

WORKOUT 64 | Dates Completed

50 lengths:
   9 crawl
 + 1/2 fly
 + 1/2 fly K
   (x5)

50 total

High-Range Lap-Swimming Workouts

These workouts of 50 to 70 lengths should take a rough minimum of 25 to 35 minutes for the fastest fitness swimmers, longer for most others. In this range, your workouts will be mostly con- tinuous swims. You'll rest only because you want to, not because you need to. Even if you're not in this range all the time, you may find it challenging to step up to these workouts and distances from time to time.

WORKOUT 65	Dates Completed		
50 lengths mixer with every 5th length K, no kickboard			
50 total			

WORKOUT 66	Dates Completed		
20 lengths crawl			
10 lengths:			
2 breast			
+ 2 back			
+ 2 breast			
+ 2 back			
+ 2 breast			
20 lengths crawl			
50 total			

WORKOUT 67	Dates Completed		
4 lengths easy			
16 lengths strokes only, no crawl			
32 lengths crawl only			
52 total			

WORKOUT 68	Dates Completed		
8 lengths P crawl			
16 lengths, all with fins:			
4 fly K			
+ 1 fly S			
+ 4 back K			
+ 1 back S			
+ 4 crawl K			
+ 2 crawl S			
24 lengths crawl			
4 lengths easy			
52 total			

WORKOUT 69	Dates Completed		
18 lengths P crawl with hand paddles			
18 lengths fin K mixer			
18 lengths strokes only, no crawl			
54 total			

WORKOUT 70	Dates Completed		
24 lengths mixer			
16 lengths:			
2 P back			
+ 2 P breast			
+ 4 P crawl			
(x2)			
8 lengths, all fin K:			
2 fly			
+ 2 back			
+ 2 crawl			
+ 2 fly			
4 lengths crawl, breathe to weakest side			
2 lengths easy			
54 total			

WORKOUT 71	Dates Completed		

7 lengths:
  ½ K + ½ water jogging
  (x7)			

14 lengths crawl			
7 lengths back			
7 lengths breast			
14 lengths crawl			

7 lengths:
  ½ water jogging + ½ elementary back
  (x7)			

56 total			

WORKOUT 72	Dates Completed		
10 lengths crawl			
9 lengths strokes only			
8 lengths crawl			
7 lengths breast			
6 lengths crawl			
5 lengths back			
4 lengths crawl			
3 lengths elementary back			
2 lengths crawl faster			
1 length fly K			
1 length water jogging			
56 total			

WORKOUT 73	Dates Completed		
18 lengths P crawl with hand paddles			
18 lengths:			
1 K			
+ 1 stroke			
(x9)			
18 lengths crawl			
4 lengths easy			
58 total			

WORKOUT 74	Dates Completed		
10 lengths crawl			
4 lengths FM			
10 lengths crawl			
4 lengths FM			
10 lengths crawl			
4 lengths FM			
10 lengths crawl			
4 lengths FM			
2 lengths easy			
58 total			

WORKOUT 75	Dates Completed		
20 lengths breast			
30 lengths crawl			
10 lengths on your back			
60 total			

WORKOUT 76	Dates Completed		
60 lengths crawl with every 10th length alternated fly K, back K, and breast K, no kickboard			
60 total			

WORKOUT 77

	Dates Completed		
20 lengths crawl			
10 lengths on your back			
20 lengths crawl			
10 lengths breast			
2 lengths easy			
62 total			

WORKOUT 78

	Dates Completed		
24 lengths crawl			
12 lengths:			
4 fly with fins			
+ 4 back with fins			
+ 4 breast			
24 lengths:			
8 P crawl			
+ 8 K crawl			
+ 8 S crawl with flip turns			
2 lengths easy			
62 total			

WORKOUT 79	Dates Completed		
64 lengths:			
4 on your back			
+ 4 breast			
+ 8 crawl			
(x4)			
64 total			

WORKOUT 80	Dates Completed		
4 lengths P crawl easy			
8 lengths breast			
12 lengths K with fins			
1 R			
+ 1 L			
(x6)			
16 lengths:			
2 crawl			
+ 1 back			
+ 1 elementary back			
(x4)			
12 lengths P crawl with hand paddles			
8 lengths FM			
4 lengths P crawl easy			
64 total			

WORKOUT 81	Dates Completed		
4 lengths easy			
25 lengths stroke mixer, no crawl			
8 lengths K, no fins			
25 lengths crawl			
4 lengths easy			
66 total			

WORKOUT 82	Dates Completed		
66 lengths crawl			
66 total			

WORKOUT 83	Dates Completed		
8 lengths any stroke			
12 lengths something completely different			
16 lengths something completely different			
28 lengths something completely different			
4 lengths something completely different			
68 total			

WORKOUT 84	Dates Completed		
4 lengths elementary back			
8 lengths fin K fly			
16 lengths crawl			
8 lengths fin K back			
4 lengths elementary back			
16 lengths crawl			
8 lengths fin K crawl			
4 lengths elementary back			
68 total			

WORKOUT 85	Dates Completed		

5 lengths:
  ½ K + ½ water jogging
  (x5)
10 lengths breast
20 lengths crawl
20 lengths breast
10 lengths crawl
 5 lengths on your back
_____
70 total			

WORKOUT 86	Dates Completed		

70 lengths:
  7 crawl
+ 1 back
+ 1 breast
+ 1 elementary back
  (x7)
_____
70 total			

Highest-Range Lap-Swimming Workouts

These workouts of 70 lengths or more should take a rough minimum of 35 to 50 minutes for the fastest fitness swimmers, and longer for most others. There are a few swimmers who do a mile or more every time they swim; these workouts reflect a deep commitment in terms of time and distances. A mile is 70 lengths.

WORKOUT 87	Dates Completed		
70 lengths all the same stroke the whole way: all back or all breast or all elementary back or all fly			
70 total			

WORKOUT 88	Dates Completed		
70 lengths crawl			
70 total			

WORKOUT 89	Dates Completed		
70 lengths crawl with every 10th length fly			
70 total			

WORKOUT 90	Dates Completed		
70 lengths all crawl:			
8 breathe regular + 2 breathe alternate sides			
+ 7 regular + 3 alternate sides			
+ 6 regular + 4 alternate sides			
+ 5 regular + 5 alternate sides			
+ 4 regular + 6 alternate sides			
+ 3 regular + 7 alternate sides			
+ 2 regular + 8 alternate sides			
70 total			

WORKOUT 91	Dates Completed		
48 lengths crawl			
24 lengths stroke mixer, no crawl			
8 lengths easy			
80 total			

WORKOUT 92	Dates Completed		
20 lengths any stroke			
40 lengths something completely different			
20 lengths something completely different			
80 total			

WORKOUT 93	Dates Completed		
80 lengths:			
4 crawl			
+4 elementary back			
+4 breast			
+4 back			
+4 crawl			
(x4)			
80 total			

WORKOUT 94	Dates Completed		
32 lengths P crawl			
24 lengths stroke and K mixer			
16 lengths P crawl:			
1 R			
+1 L			
+2 regular			
(x4)			
8 lengths:			
1 back			
+1 elementary back			
(x4)			
80 total			

WORKOUT 95	Dates Completed		
6 lengths easy			
12 lengths fin K			
24 lengths stroke mixer, no crawl			
48 lengths crawl			
90 total			

WORKOUT 96	Dates Completed		
15 lengths stroke mixer, no crawl			
30 lengths crawl			
15 lengths stroke mixer, no crawl			
30 lengths S crawl with fins			
90 total			

WORKOUT 97	Dates Completed		
30 lengths P crawl			
15 lengths fin K			
30 lengths:			
10 back			
+ 10 breast			
+ 10 elementary back			
15 lengths, all easy crawl:			
5 P			
+ 5 K			
+ 5 S			
90 total			

WORKOUT 98	Dates Completed		
10 lengths stroke mixer, no crawl			
30 lengths crawl			
10 lengths fin K mixer			
30 lengths crawl			
10 lengths easy			
90 total			

WORKOUT 99

	Dates Completed		
6 lengths easy			
40 lengths P crawl with hand paddles			
12 lengths fin K			
40 lengths S crawl with fins			
2 lengths easy			
100 total			

WORKOUT 100

	Dates Completed		
4 lengths easy			
16 lengths stroke mixer, no crawl			
48 lengths crawl			
32 lengths:			
1 P crawl			
+ 1 K crawl			
+ 2 S			
(x8)			
100 total			

WORKOUT 101	Dates Completed		
6 lengths easy			
24 lengths back			
40 lengths crawl:			
20 slow			
+ 20 faster			
24 lengths breast			
6 lengths easy			
100 total			

WORKOUT 102	Dates Completed		
100 lengths all crawl			
100 total			

SIX

Other Workout Formats

THE WORKOUT FORMATS in this chapter go beyond lap swimming and provide even more variety in how to organize and complete your fitness-swimming workouts.

Timed Workouts

In timed workouts, the variable is the number of minutes you swim. You can swim different lengths of time on different days. While doing these workouts, do not count lengths or laps; think about something else as you swim. You can use a regular clock, a pace clock, a wristwatch, or a stopwatch to time your sets. Don't be obsessive about the timing, however—just get as close to the time period of the set as you can.

WORKOUT 103	Dates Completed		
4 minutes on your back			
6 minutes breast			
8 minutes crawl			
2 minutes water jogging			
20 minutes total			

WORKOUT 104	Dates Completed		
6 minutes crawl			
1 minute back			
6 minutes crawl			
1 minute breast			
6 minutes crawl			
1 minute elementary back			
21 minutes total			

WORKOUT 105	Dates Completed		
1 minute easy			
3 minutes crawl, breathing to strong side			
7 minutes crawl, breathing to weak side			
11 minutes crawl, breathing to alternate sides			
22 minutes total			

WORKOUT 106	Dates Completed		
1 minute elementary back			
10 minutes back			
1 minute fly K			
10 minutes breast			
1 minute water jogging			
23 minutes total			

WORKOUT 107	Dates Completed		
8 minutes mixer			
12 minutes crawl			
4 minutes elementary back			
24 minutes total			

WORKOUT 108	Dates Completed		
5 minutes P			
15 minutes mixer			
5 minutes K			
25 minutes total			

WORKOUT 109

	Dates Completed		

2 minutes water jogging
4 minutes crawl, breathing to alternate sides
8 minutes fin K on sides and back
12 minutes crawl, breathing to weak side

26 minutes total

WORKOUT 110

	Dates Completed		

3 minutes fin K on R
9 minutes choice
12 minutes crawl
3 minutes fin K on L

27 minutes total

SHELBYVILLE-SHELBY COUNTY
PUBLIC LIBRARY

WORKOUT 111	Dates Completed		
4 minutes K with fins			
8 minutes P crawl R–L			
4 minutes stroke mixer, no crawl			
8 minutes crawl			
4 minutes K, no fins			
28 minutes total			

WORKOUT 112	Dates Completed		
9 minutes crawl			
1 minute fly			
9 minutes crawl			
1 minute fly			
9 minutes crawl			
29 minutes total			

WORKOUT 113	Dates Completed		
30 minutes mixer			
30 minutes total			

WORKOUT 114	Dates Completed		
1 minute water jogging			
30 minutes all back or all breast or all elementary back			
31 minutes total			

WORKOUT 115

	Dates Completed		

10 minutes crawl
 5 minutes on your back
10 minutes crawl
 5 minutes breast
 2 minutes easy
_____
32 minutes total

WORKOUT 116

	Dates Completed		

 9 minutes P crawl
 6 minutes strokes
 3 minutes fin K
 6 minutes strokes
 9 minutes crawl
_____
33 minutes total

WORKOUT 117	Dates Completed		
2 minutes easy			
6 minutes S fly with fins			
18 minutes crawl			
6 minutes S back with fins			
2 minutes easy			
34 minutes total			

WORKOUT 118	Dates Completed		
2½ minutes K			
7½ minutes on your back			
15 minutes crawl			
7½ minutes breast			
2½ minutes K			
35 minutes total			

WORKOUT 119	Dates Completed		
20 minutes stroke mixer, no crawl			
10 minutes crawl			
5 minutes K			
1 minute easy			
36 minutes total			

WORKOUT 120	Dates Completed		
25 minutes crawl			
12 minutes any other stroke			
37 minutes total			

WORKOUT 121	Dates Completed		
5 minutes fin K			
14 minutes P crawl R–L			
14 minutes crawl			
5 minutes K			
38 minutes total			

WORKOUT 122	Dates Completed		
15 minutes breast			
13 minutes on your back			
11 minutes choice			
39 minutes total			

WORKOUT 123	Dates Completed		
10 minutes on your back			
20 minutes P crawl			
10 minutes breast			
40 minutes total			

WORKOUT 124	Dates Completed		
4 minutes easy			
8 minutes fin K			
12 minutes P crawl with hand paddles			
16 minutes stroke mixer, no crawl			
1 minute easy			
41 minutes total			

WORKOUT 125

	Dates Completed		

 7 minutes crawl
14 minutes choice
21 minutes crawl
————————————
42 minutes total

WORKOUT 126

	Dates Completed		

 2 minutes water jogging
40 minutes crawl
 1 minute elementary back
————————————
43 minutes total

WORKOUT 127

	Dates Completed	

11 minutes breast
22 minutes crawl
11 minutes on your back

44 minutes total

WORKOUT 128

	Dates Completed	

15 minutes P, all strokes
15 minutes fin K, all strokes
15 minutes crawl with flip turns on deep-end wall

45 minutes total

Pattern Workouts

These workouts combine elements of lap swimming and timed workouts. You follow a repeating pattern for however long you want to swim. Follow the pattern listed as many times as possible for whatever time period you choose on any given day.

WORKOUT 129	Dates Completed		

Use this pattern for _____ minutes:
    1 length crawl
  + 1 length stroke . . .			

WORKOUT 130	Dates Completed		

Use this pattern for _____ minutes:
    2 lengths stroke
  + 1 length crawl . . .			

WORKOUT 131	Dates Completed		

Use this pattern for _____ minutes:
    1 length fly K
  + 3 lengths breast
  + 2 lengths back
  + 1 length elementary back . . .			

WORKOUT 132	Dates Completed		

Use this pattern for _____ minutes:
    2 lengths crawl
  + 4 lengths stroke
  + 1 breast
  + 1 back
  + 1 breast
  + 1 elementary back . . .			

WORKOUT 133	Dates Completed		
Use this pattern for _____ minutes:			
6 lengths crawl			
+ 3 lengths stroke			
+ 1 length fly K . . .			

WORKOUT 134	Dates Completed		
Use this pattern for _____ minutes:			
4 lengths crawl			
+ 2 lengths stroke . . .			

WORKOUT 135	Dates Completed		
Use this pattern for _____ minutes: 　　7　lengths crawl 　+ 3　lengths breast . . .			

WORKOUT 136	Dates Completed		
Use this pattern for _____ minutes: 　　5　lengths crawl with flip turns 　+ 1　length fly K with hands held together 　　　behind back . . .			

WORKOUT 137

Dates Completed

Use this pattern for _____ minutes:

    8 lengths P crawl with hand paddles
+ 4 lengths fin K . . .

WORKOUT 138

Dates Completed

Use this pattern for _____ minutes:

    10 lengths crawl
+ 5 lengths stroke . . .

WORKOUT 139

Dates Completed

Use this pattern for _____ minutes:

    8 lengths crawl
+ 4 lengths stroke
+ 2 lengths K . . .

WORKOUT 140

Dates Completed

Use this pattern for _____ minutes:

    2 lengths breast
+ 1 length water jogging
+ 2 lengths crawl
+ 1 length water jogging
+ 2 lengths elementary back . . .

WORKOUT 141	Dates Completed		
Use this pattern for _____ minutes:			
3 lengths crawl			
+2 lengths breast			
+1 length on your back . . .			

WORKOUT 142	Dates Completed		
Use this pattern for _____ minutes:			
6 lengths strokes:			
2 back			
+2 breast			
+2 elementary back			
+3 lengths crawl:			
1 breathe R			
+1 breathe L			
+1 breathing alternate sides			
+1 length K . . .			

WORKOUT 143	Dates Completed		
Use this pattern for _____ minutes:			
3 lengths crawl			
+ 1 length breast, right arm only			
+ 3 lengths crawl			
+ 1 length breast, left arm only . . .			

WORKOUT 144	Dates Completed		
Use this pattern for _____ minutes:			
1 length crawl			
+ 1 length stroke			
+ 1 length crawl			
+ 1 length K . . .			

WORKOUT 145	Dates Completed		
Use this pattern for _____ minutes:			
4 lengths breast			
+ 1 length fly K			
+ 4 lengths alternating back and			
elementary back			
+ 1 length fly K . . .			

WORKOUT 146	Dates Completed		
Use this pattern for _____ minutes:			
1 length back			
+ 1 length crawl R			
+ 1 length breast			
+ 1 length crawl L			
+ 1 length elementary back			
+ 1 length crawl breathing alternate sides . . .			

WORKOUT 147	Dates Completed		
Use this pattern for _____ minutes:			
1 length crawl			
+ 1 length breast			
+ 2 lengths crawl			
+ 2 lengths breast			
+ 3 lengths crawl			
+ 3 lengths breast			
(keep building)			

WORKOUT 148	Dates Completed		
Use this pattern for _____ minutes:			
6 lengths crawl			
+ 5 lengths breast			
+ 4 lengths crawl			
+ 3 lengths back			
+ 2 lengths crawl			
+ 1 length elementary back . . .			

WORKOUT 149	Dates Completed		
Use this pattern for _____ minutes:			
2 lengths crawl			
+ 1 length crawl R			
+ 1 length crawl L			
+ 2 lengths breast			
+ 1 length breast R			
+ 1 length breast L			
+ 1 length elementary back . . .			

WORKOUT 150	Dates Completed		
Use this pattern for _____ minutes:			
10 lengths crawl:			
1 breathe R			
+ 1 breathe L			
+ 2 breathe R			
+ 2 breathe L			
+ 4 breathe alternate sides			
+ 2 lengths stroke or K . . .			

WORKOUT 151	Dates Completed		
Use this pattern for _____ minutes: 1 length crawl + 1 length back + 1 length breast + 1 length elementary back + 2 lengths crawl + 2 lengths back + 2 lengths breast + 2 lengths elementary back . . . (keep building)			

WORKOUT 152	Dates Completed		
Use this pattern for _____ minutes: 1 length crawl + 1 length back + 1 length breast + 1 length elementary back + 2 lengths P crawl R-L + 2 lengths crawl + 2 lengths back + 2 lengths breast + 2 lengths elementary back + 2 lengths P crawl R-L . . .			

WORKOUT 153

	Dates Completed	

Use this pattern for _____ minutes:

    1 length crawl + 1 length stroke
+ 2 lengths crawl + 1 length stroke
+ 3 lengths crawl + 1 length stroke
+ 4 lengths crawl + 1 length stroke
+ 5 lengths crawl + 1 length stroke
+ 6 lengths crawl + 1 length stroke
(keep building)

WORKOUT 154

	Dates Completed	

Use this pattern for _____ minutes:

    3 lengths on your back
+ 2 lengths breast
+ 1 length crawl . . .

Mixed Workouts
Each mixed workout contains at least
one lap-swim set and one timed set.

WORKOUT 155	Dates Completed		
10 minutes stroke mixer, no crawl			
20 lengths crawl			

WORKOUT 156	Dates Completed		
10 lengths breast			
10 minutes crawl			
10 lengths on your back			

WORKOUT 157	Dates Completed		
32 lengths P crawl			
8 minutes breast			

WORKOUT 158	Dates Completed		
6 minutes crawl			
12 lengths stroke mixer, no crawl			
6 minutes:			
3 K			
+ 3 easy			

WORKOUT 159	Dates Completed		
4 minutes stroke mixer, no crawl			
8 lengths crawl			
8 minutes fin K			
8 lengths:			
1 stroke			
+ 1 water jogging			
(x4)			
2 minutes crawl			

WORKOUT 160	Dates Completed		
12 lengths crawl			
12 minutes on your back			
12 lengths crawl			

WORKOUT 161	Dates Completed		
2½ minutes easy			
30 lengths crawl			
5 minutes fin K on your back			

WORKOUT 162	Dates Completed		
5 minutes K with board			
10 lengths elementary back			
5 minutes K, no board			
10 lengths breast			

WORKOUT 163	Dates Completed		
8 lengths easy			
12 minutes weakest stroke (no crawl)			
16 lengths crawl			

WORKOUT 164	Dates Completed		
4 lengths easy			
8 minutes stroke and K mixer			
4 lengths easy			
8 minutes crawl			
4 lengths easy			

WORKOUT 165	Dates Completed		
8 minutes crawl			
16 lengths on your back			
4 minutes breast			
4 lengths easy			

WORKOUT 166	Dates Completed		
5 minutes stroke mixer, no crawl			
20 lengths crawl			
5 minutes fin K fly on your back			
10 lengths crawl			

WORKOUT 167	Dates Completed		
16 lengths crawl			
8 minutes breast			
16 lengths crawl			
4 minutes K			

WORKOUT 168	Dates Completed		
20 lengths crawl			
5 minutes on your back			
10 lengths crawl			
5 minutes easy			

WORKOUT 169	Dates Completed		
10 minutes R-L strokes only			
20 lengths crawl breathing to alternate sides			
5 minutes fin K			

WORKOUT 170	Dates Completed		
20 lengths mixer			
10 minutes back or breast			
10 lengths mixer			
5 minutes elementary back			

WORKOUT 171	Dates Completed		
3 minutes P crawl			
30 lengths mixer			
3 minutes K crawl			

WORKOUT 172	Dates Completed		
5 minutes crawl			
10 lengths stroke and K mixer			
5 minutes P crawl R-L			
10 lengths all one stroke			
5 minutes crawl			

WORKOUT 173	Dates Completed		
5 minutes easy			
40 lengths crawl			
2½ minutes easy			

WORKOUT 174	Dates Completed		
20 lengths P crawl with hand paddles			
10 minutes all one stroke			
5 lengths easy			

WORKOUT 175	Dates Completed		
10 minutes mixer			
20 lengths crawl breathing to best side			
2½ minutes water jogging			
10 lengths crawl breathing to weak side			
5 minutes mixer			

WORKOUT 176	Dates Completed		
10 lengths stroke mixer, no crawl			
5 minutes P crawl with hand paddles			
20 lengths crawl			
5 minutes fin K fly			

WORKOUT 177	Dates Completed		
15 minutes P crawl with hand paddles			
20 lengths breast or on your back			
5 minutes fin K on your sides			

WORKOUT 178	Dates Completed		
16 minutes mixer			
8 lengths:			
4 best stroke			
+4 worst stroke (no crawl)			
4 minutes water jogging			

WORKOUT 179	Dates Completed		
7½ minutes warm-up			
25 lengths crawl			
2½ minutes warm-down			

Short Timed Workouts

The variable in these workouts again is time; the idea is to swim as far as possible to fill the given time periods. If you've grown tired of always counting lengths or laps, try timed-format workouts, either these short ones or the longer ones given earlier. Then you'll be free to concentrate on other things while you swim. Time your sets with some type of clock or watch.

The short workouts that follow are good starter workouts for beginning fitness swimmers. They also can serve as easier workouts if you're on a hard–easy workout cycle, or you can use a short workout if you have a time restriction on a particular day and can't do your normal distance or time.

We tend to think of exercise in "all or none" terms—that is, either we're on a full-scale training program or we don't exercise at all. Perhaps a reduced-duration program, such as these 10- to 20-minute timed swimming workouts, could be a useful option at times in your personal fitness workouts. Some exercise is better than none.

WORKOUT 180	Dates Completed		
2 minutes crawl			
4 minutes on your back			
3 minutes breast			
1 minute crawl			
10 minutes total			

WORKOUT 181	Dates Completed		
10 minutes stroke mixer, no crawl			
10 minutes total			

WORKOUT 182	Dates Completed		
1 minute easy			
4 minutes crawl			
3 minutes K, no board, no fins			
2 minutes crawl			
1 minute easy			
11 minutes total			

WORKOUT 183	Dates Completed		
1 minute easy			
3 minutes P crawl R-L			
3 minutes fin K crawl R-L			
3 minutes crawl			
1 minute easy			
11 minutes total			

WORKOUT 184

	Dates Completed		
6 minutes P crawl			
3 minutes fin K fly			
2 minutes breast			
1 minute easy			
12 minutes total			

WORKOUT 185

	Dates Completed		
4 minutes on your back			
4 minutes breast			
4 minutes crawl			
12 minutes total			

WORKOUT 186	Dates Completed		
5 minutes P crawl with hand paddles			
7 minutes fin K fly and crawl on your sides			
1 minute easy			
13 minutes total			

WORKOUT 187	Dates Completed		
2 minutes easy			
4 minutes			
1 K			
+ 1 stroke			
(x2)			
6 minutes crawl breathing to alternate sides			
1 minute easy			
13 minutes total			

WORKOUT 188	Dates Completed		
1 minute easy			
3 minutes:			
1 back			
+ 1 breast			
+ 1 elementary back			
6 minutes crawl			
3 minutes fin K back			
1 minute easy			
14 minutes total			

WORKOUT 189	Dates Completed		
8 minutes P			
4 minutes K			
2 minutes S			
14 minutes total			

WORKOUT 190	Dates Completed		
3 minutes crawl			
5 minutes K, no fins, no board			
7 minutes stroke mixer, no crawl			
15 minutes total			

WORKOUT 191	Dates Completed		
3 minutes easy P			
3 minutes crawl			
3 minutes elementary back			
3 minutes crawl			
3 minutes easy K			
15 minutes total			

WORKOUT 192	Dates Completed		
1 minute easy P			
2 minutes elementary back			
3 minutes breast			
4 minutes back			
5 minutes crawl			
1 minute easy K			
16 minutes total			

WORKOUT 193	Dates Completed		
2 minutes breast			
3 minutes P crawl R-L			
6 minutes crawl			
3 minutes P crawl R-L			
2 minutes on your back			
16 minutes total			

WORKOUT 194	Dates Completed		
8 minutes P crawl with hand paddles			
5 minutes fin K on your sides			
3 minutes crawl with flip turns			
1 minute easy			
17 minutes total			

WORKOUT 195	Dates Completed		
1 minute easy			
3 minutes fin K fly on your back			
5 minutes all one stroke			
8 minutes crawl			
17 minutes total			

WORKOUT 196 | Dates Completed

2 minutes P
6 minutes on your back
2 minutes K
6 minutes breast
2 minutes easy

18 minutes total

WORKOUT 197 | Dates Completed

3 minutes P crawl
6 minutes fin K crawl
9 minutes crawl with flip turns on
    shallow-end wall

18 minutes total

WORKOUT 198	Dates Completed		
2 minutes warm-up			
16 minutes P crawl breathing to weak side only			
1 minute warm-down			
19 minutes total			

WORKOUT 199	Dates Completed		
7 minutes P crawl			
2 minutes S fly with fins			
7 minutes P crawl			
2 minutes S fly with fins			
1 minute easy			
19 minutes total			

WORKOUT 200	Dates Completed		
8 minutes crawl			
6 minutes:			
1 back			
+ 1 breast			
(x3)			
4 minutes fin K fly on front, both sides, and back			
2 minutes P elementary back			
20 minutes total			

WORKOUT 201	Dates Completed		
20 minutes mixer			
20 minutes total			

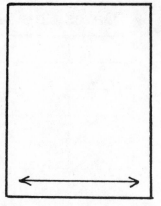

Swim widths (30 feet here).

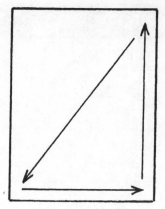

Swim triangles.

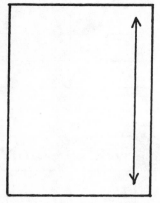

Swim lengths (40 feet here).

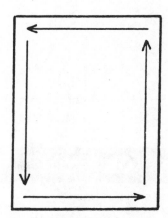

Swim rectangles.

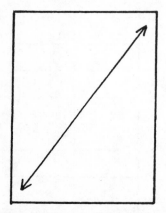

Swim diagonals (50 feet here).

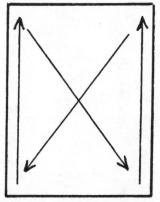

Swim side walls and diagonals.

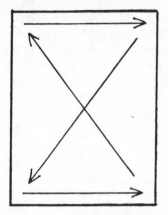

Swim end walls and diagonals.

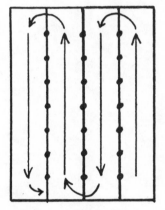

Swim snake in lanes.

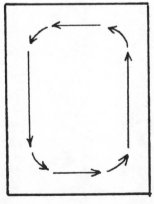

Swim circle without touching.

Fitness Swimming in Small Pools

Not every pool is regulation length. Travelers often encounter small pools at hotels. There's no reason to interrupt your fitness routine if, for a few days, you don't have access to a regular pool. In fact, swimming in a small pool is a great way to add variety to your fitness-swimming workouts.

Our Aquatics Center includes a separate 30-by-40-foot diving area, which is not used most of the time. When no one is diving, our swimmers sometimes use the diving tank.

You can mix up strokes, kicks, pulls, and so on for the whole patterns described below, or you can do different things for different lengths and widths of your workout.

You'll have to decide whether to work your turns and push-offs strong or to go easy in these short distances. You'll need to improvise a little with your hand touches and foot placement to keep yourself going in the right direction. Be a little cautious doing the back stroke, since most diving areas do not have back stroke flags.

Some very basic patterns are outlined here for your use:

You can swim sequences, combining some of the basic patterns shown above. For example, alternate "rectangles" and "end walls and diagonals" throughout your workout.

You can create even more variety by tracing letter patterns as you swim. Swim forward and backward along the letter shape, using lengths, widths, and diagonals. The letters *L, M, N, V. U,* and *Z* are good ones to swim.

These workouts give you a chance to skip counting laps. Just follow the pattern for a certain amount of time, such as 20 or 30 minutes.

Swimming in a confined space, such as a diving area or cross-pool, is the opposite of long-course training (in a 50-meter pool), another useful variation. Occasionally performing workouts as described above will help you prolong your longevity as a fitness swimmer.

SEVEN

More Workout Variations

BEYOND THE SUBSETS listed in the previous workouts, there are many other procedures and pieces of equipment that you can use from time to time to keep your total fitness-swimming program fun and interesting.

Running in the Water

Water jogging, or running in shallow water, is not exactly swimming, but it is a procedure you can use occasionally to do something different in the pool. For the best effect, the water should be between waist-deep and chest-deep. The water will support most of your body weight, reducing much of the impact when your feet strike the pool bottom. The pool bottom may be slippery, but you'll quickly adjust and be able to run without falling. Use water jogging to break up a long swim or as part of your warm-up or warm-down. The main variations are running forward, backward, sideways to the right or left ("side hops"), and sideways to the right or left crossing the legs over front and back alternately.

You can run laps around the deep end of the pool, provided you are supported by a water-ski vest, an innertube, a swim bubble, a rescue tube, a Wet Vest, or an Aqua Jogger. These devices keep your head out of water while the rest of you is submerged to neck level. They permit you to lean forward slightly and simulate a true running style in the water. Move your arms as if you were running and not swimming. Underwater, you need length or reach to your stride (no baby steps), going easy on the forward stroke and stronger on the backward action. Lean into the run just a little. Expect very slow movement in the water in comparison with running on land or swimming. A standard program of deep-water running might be for 10 to 20 minutes.

In a small pool, you can tether yourself

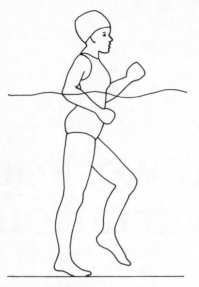

You can use water jogging on the pool bottom for variety in warm-up and warm-down routines or to break up long swims.

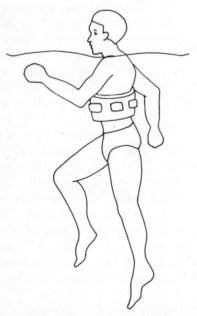

The key to water running is to go easy on the forward stroke and stronger on the backward action.

so that you're running in place. You may want to play music on the poolside to help keep this procedure appealing. Use sensible safety precautions with electrical devices near water.

In addition to being unusual procedures for fitness swimmers, water jogging and deep-water running are often used by runners to maintain fitness while rehabilitating an injury (hydrotherapy) or to supplement their running training program. The origins of these procedures can be traced back to veterinary medicine and the common practice of exercising racehorses in troughs or pools of water for therapy.

Water Exercises

Water exercises are calisthenics and stretches in the water. Entire fitness programs, for those who do not wish to swim, are built around this concept. The water provides its own extra resistance to these hydroaerobic exercises and promotes good muscular stretching and joint flexibility (especially if the water is warm enough). These types of exercises can be done slowly to develop flexibility, or fast and continuously to add in the cardiovascular factor. Music and choreography are often used to maintain a fast cadence and up-tempo attitude.

Just as with calisthenics on land, you can accommodate quickly to these water exercises. As you adjust, you may need to do more repetitions or spend more time on each exercise. You may get bored if you do a small number of exercises over and over, however, so keep variety in your program. You can start with ten repetitions on most of the moving exercises or with 10 seconds on the static stretches, and then build up. There are hundreds of exercises you can do.

Fitness with Your Head Up

There are some people who would like to exercise in the water but haven't mastered breathing or don't want to get their faces wet. There's a surprising amount that you can do in the water with your face or head up. The following are some ideas:

• Water jogging on the pool bottom, along with deep-water running, and water exercises plus walk laps on the pool bottom (water walking).

• Kick with a kickboard, with or without fins. Crawl kick on your front, back, or sides. Fly kick on your front, back, or sides.

• Breast stroke with your head up, back stroke, elementary back stroke, or even side stroke.

• Tread water in deep water. Use your hands or hold your hands up.

• Use a pull buoy and hold one or two kickboards under one arm for one-arm pulling. Use the right arm only down the pool and the left arm only back.

• Fin kick with a kickboard for one-leg kicking. Use the right leg only down the pool and the left leg only back.

• Pull breast stroke while suspended inside an innertube, or pull crawl or fly while lying on a small surfboard.

Mixing Up Your Strokes

There are many different ways to practice a stroke beyond just swimming the stroke. Use the following lists to create many different subsets in your workouts in terms of the basic fitness-swimming strokes.

CRAWL.
Pull with pull buoy (P).
Pull with hand paddles.
Pull with one arm only (R-L).

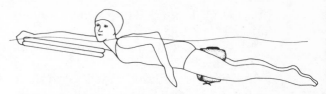

One-arm pulling with head up is one of the many exercises that you can do without getting your face wet.

Pull with fist swimming (hands clenched).

Pull while holding a tennis ball in each hand.

Pull a partner who holds your ankles and kicks a little.

Kick with or without a kickboard (K).

Kick with your arms overhead, by your sides, or out at shoulder level.

Kick with your hands behind your back or out in front and with your head up.

Kick on your sides (R-L).

Kick with a series of full twists.

Kick on the surface or underwater.

Kick with or without fins.

Swim with your head up.

Swim with fins.

Try different breathing patterns—to right side only or left side only every stroke or every other stroke; every third stroke alternated to opposite sides; two to the right and two to the left; four or more to the right and four or more to the left; every fifth stroke alternated to opposite sides; swim a very short distance without breathing.

BACK STROKE.
Pull with pull buoy (P).
Pull with double-arm back stroke.
Pull with hand paddles.
Pull with fist swimming (hands clenched).

Pull while holding a tennis ball in each hand.

Pull a partner who holds your ankles and kicks a little.

Kick with or without a kickboard (K).

Kick with your arms by your sides, overhead, out at shoulder level, or straight up in the air.

Kick with your hands behind your back or on top of your head, or with your elbows in by your sides and your hands straight up.

Kick with or without fins.

Swim with one arm only (R-L).

Swim with a definite stopping of each hand by the hip before lifting it into the recovery.

Swim with a definite continuous hand action, moving each hand past the hip and swinging up into the recovery in one smooth action.

Swim with fins.

Swim with exaggerated body or shoulder roll.

BREAST STROKE.

Pull with pull buoy (P).

Pull with hand paddles.

Pull with fist (hands clenched).

Pull while holding a tennis ball in each hand.

Pull while suspended inside an innertube.

Kick with or without a kickboard (K).

Kick with the hands stretched backward, touching the fingertips to the heels or ankles during each kick.

Kick with the hands stretched out in front of the shoulders, breathing after two or three kicks.

Kick on your back—inverted breast stroke kick.

Kick while treading water in deep water; try this while holding your thumbs up, or try lifting your shoulders and chest up above the surface of the water (use your hands, too).

Swim with your head up.

Swim with one arm only (R-L).

Swim with a double pull (breathing every other stroke) and compare with breathing every stroke.

Swim with an exaggerated glide forward every stroke.

ELEMENTARY BACK STROKE.

Pull with a pull buoy (P).

Pull with hand paddles.

Pull with fist (hands clenched).

Pull while holding a tennis ball in each hand.

Pull a partner who holds your ankles and kicks a little.

Kick with or without a kickboard (K).

Kick with your arms by your sides, overhead, out at shoulder level, or straight up in the air.

Kick with your hands behind your back or on top of your head, or with your elbows in by your sides and your hands straight up.

Swim with one arm only (R-L).

Swim and count your strokes for 1 length; work to lower your count by stroking stronger and gliding farther.

Swim with an exaggerated glide every stroke.

BUTTERFLY.

Pull with pull buoy (P).

Pull with hand paddles.

Pull with fist swimming (hands clenched).

Pull while holding a tennis ball in each hand.

Kick with or without a kickboard (K).

Kick underwater or on the surface.

Kick on your front, sides, or back.

Kick with or without fins.

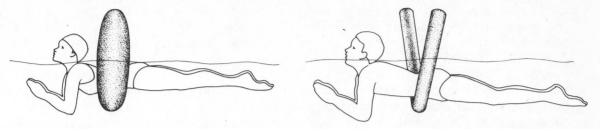

A regular car-tire innertube or a woggle can help with your breast stroke practice.

Swim with fins.

Swim with one arm only (R-L).

Swim on your back with the fly kick and the double overarm stroke.

Try different breathing patterns—every stroke, every second stroke, every third stroke, or a very short distance without breathing.

INNERTUBES AND SURFBOARDS.

Car-tire-size innertubes can be used with breast stroke pull in the water. Our tubes are 13 inches inside diameter, but larger tubes will work as well. Lie with the upper part of your stomach, just below the rib cage, inside the tube to practice the breast stroke arm action. Be careful not to poke or scratch yourself if the tube has a protruding valve stem.

Keep your head up, and don't kick—just work on the arm stroke. Concentrate on a wide, circular pull. Go through a full range of motion, reaching far forward with your hands but not coming back beyond shoulder level with the upper arms or elbows (never touch the tube).

If you feel lower back pain while lying in the tube, bend your knees and hips a little to flatten out your back, but don't arch. If you tilt forward when you pull or if it's hard to keep your forearms in the water, readjust your position in the tube or deflate the tube slightly.

You can use a device called a woggle, available at pool supply stores, instead of an innertube to practice your breast stroke pull. Lie across this foam cylinder, which is about 3 inches in diameter and 66 inches long.

A Styrofoam surfboard about 4 feet by 15 inches can be purchased during the summer at most toy stores. Lie on this to practice the crawl and butterfly arm strokes. Although initially it's tricky to keep your balance, concentrate on the propulsive parts of these strokes, being strong on the underwater pull and easy on the recovery. Focus on distance per stroke, getting the most out of each stroke by creating the greatest forward movement with each arm pull. Keep your chin on the board, look forward, and do not kick. Do not use this proce-

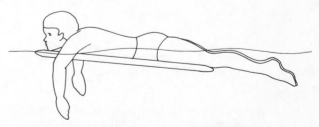

For crawl and butterfly stroke practice, lie on a Styrofoam surfboard.

dure, however, if you experience any severe shoulder pain during or after the pulling.

WEIGHTED DEVICES. Wrist weights are ¼- to 1-pound weights worn around your wrists. The added weight makes you feel your stroke better, especially in terms of rhythm, timing, and hand speed. Although wrist weights are relatively light, they help you develop muscular endurance, since you move them hundreds of times during a fitness-swimming workout. This in-the-water exercise program strengthens the actual range of motion of the arm action of the various swimming strokes. Do not use this exercise, however, if you experience any severe shoulder pain during or after the pulling.

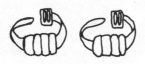

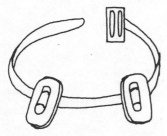

Weighted devices, like these wrist weights and scuba weight belt, help you feel the rhythm, timing, and speed of your stroke, as well as help you develop muscular endurance.

Wrist weights work best along with a pull buoy to offset the extra weight and negative buoyancy. Use mostly crawl, though you can perform any stroke. Warm up thoroughly before using the wrist weights to prepare your arms and shoulders for the extra effort. Wrist weights can also be used as ankle weights during kicking or fin kicking.

Fitness swimmers can also strap on a scuba weight belt; 2 to 8 pounds will make you work harder against the constant extra load. This will also show you just how much influence extra weight can have on your efficiency in the water. The reduction in speed due to the added weight is startling. Again, avoid this procedure if it produces shoulder pain.

Use one or two pull buoys to counterbalance the heavy negative buoyancy. Use mostly crawl, though you can perform any stroke. To prevent you from arching your back, strap the weights around both your legs and the pull buoy, or else place them very low on the hips. Strap the weights around one or two kickboards to kick or fin kick against greater resistance.

DRAG DEVICES. Drag devices create resistance to your progress through the water. There are conditioning and strengthening benefits to working harder against the increased drag on your movement through the water. When you remove the devices, you will feel smoother and faster in the water, in touch with the flow of the water over your skin as you swim.

A drag board is a flat, buoyant board with two holes into which you slide your ankles. When you assume a swimming position, the surface of the board becomes vertical in the water, creating a drag effect. You'll probably use this with a pull buoy mostly for crawl, though you can use it for other strokes as well.

A drag suit has large exterior pockets that expand and fill with water as you swim, creating a drag effect. This is a refinement of the old concept of swimming while wearing several swimsuits, a sweatsuit, or a tee shirt and gym shorts (swimming in old tennis shoes is fun, too). You can swim any stroke while wearing a drag suit without altering normal body position.

Stretch cords are made of surgical tubing (18 to 20 feet of tubing with $3/8$-inch outer diameter and $3/16$-inch inner diameter works well in a 25-yard pool). One end of this stretching tether is tied to a belt around the swimmer's waist, and the other end forms a loop to attach to a starting block. You swim to the opposite end of the pool against the increasing resistance of the stretch cord, stop briefly to turn the belt around, and then, with an assist from the strongly contracting elastic tubing, return faster than normally possible. Be sure to replace frayed tubing and never stand directly in line with the stretched-out tubing.

A regular plastic bucket can be used as a drag device in the pool. A 10-quart bucket is a good size, although 6 or 8 quarts would work well, too. Drill eight or ten $1/4$-inch holes in the bottom of the bucket to smooth out its flow as it trails behind you through the water. Attach an 8-foot rope to its handle, and tie the other end around your waist. You'll be using the crawl with a pull buoy mostly, but you can swim any of the strokes against the strong resistance of the bucket.

CROSS-POOL WORKOUTS. About once or twice a year, our pool is set up so

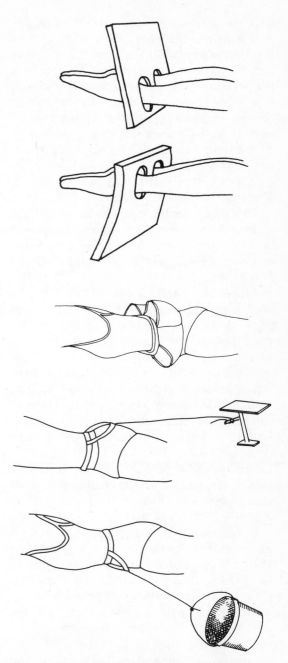

By creating more resistance in the water, drag devices (drag board, drag suit, stretching tether, and bucket) increase strengthening and conditioning.

that the lane lines run cross-pool (a 52-foot width in our case). You may have to improvise to attach the lane lines, but it can be done in most pools. Although a few swimmers are upset by this change, it becomes a fun workout for most of our fitness swimmers, promoting even more variety in their total training program.

You'll have to think a lot about converting distances to the cross-pool format. In our pool, 3 widths almost equals 2 lengths (50 yards).

When swimming cross-pool, you'll get more practice on your turns and push-offs. It can be hard to see the turns without any markings or flags, so make them carefully.

MIRRORS AND VIDEOTAPING. "To see ourselves as others see us" is the goal of using reflective mirrors in the pool. Like many popular ideas, this one is not completely new. I saw a real glass mirror used in McCurdy Natatorium when I was a freshman at Springfield College (Massachusetts) in 1965, and mirrors are commonly used in dance, ballet, and aerobic exercise classes. You can purchase a 4-by-4-foot or 4-by-8-foot mirror in order to watch yourself as you swim. The mirror should be shatterproof and have an aluminum border that keeps it flat and rigid.

In the water, the mirror can be placed at the end of the lane so that you can see yourself swimming into it, at the side of the pool so that you can see yourself in a profile view from the right or left side, or on the pool bottom so that you can see yourself swimming over the mirror.

Out of the water, the mirror can be mounted in the gutter in front of the starting block so that you can see yourself swimming into and away from it.

Another feedback system at our pool includes a videocamera with surface and underwater filming capabilities, a VCR with slow-motion capacity, and a large playback monitor—all right there in my poolside office for planned or spontaneous use. You can swim toward the camera, away from the camera, and across the camera's view (in profile from both sides). In general, there's too much surface analysis in swimming and too little underwater analysis of strokes and turns. An underwater view of strokes is most significant because this is where propulsion occurs. This procedure is like seeing yourself in a swimming textbook.

BIATHLONS AND TRIATHLONS. For those who do some running as well as swimming, the biathlon combines these two fitness activities. Although any distances can be used, a common procedure is to run 2 miles and then immediately swim ½ mile; the usual ratio is 4:1 run:swim. Other patterns include swim-run-swim or run-swim-run.

The triathlon combines the three fitness activities of swimming, biking, and running. Many combinations of distances can be created. A standard triathlon is 1.5 kilometers (0.9 mile) swim plus 40 kilometers (24.6 miles) bike plus 10 kilometers (6.2 miles) run. The Hawaiian Iron Man Contest is exceptionally long, consisting of a 2.5-mile ocean swim plus a 112-mile bike ride plus a 26.2-mile run (a full marathon).

Although these examples are competitive events or races, I'd like to challenge you to think of occasionally using the biathlon or triathlon concept as a different type of fitness workout. Presumably, you're already a good swimmer. If necessary, you could substitute walking, water jogging, or deep-water running for running, and a stationary bike for biking.

OPEN-WATER SWIMMING. There's a tremendous difference between swimming in a pool and swimming in open water. Judging distances over the water can be deceiving, and official distances are often only estimates. Constantly changing conditions affect speed and performance over the same distance on different occasions. Tides, currents, undertows, rips, waves, and marine life also affect performance, so you should learn all you can about their influences. Cold water presents another risk to the swimmer, since water conducts heat away from the body twenty-five times faster than does air of the same temperature.

Observe the following guidelines when swimming in open water to reduce risk and perform better:

• Never train or swim alone.

• Know the direction and layout of your swimming course (e.g., parallel to shore, around buoys, or straight across the lake).

• Wear a bathing cap to help retain heat (30 to 50 percent of the body's heat is lost through the head) and to help observers keep you in sight.

• Practice under cold water conditions, and know the symptoms and treatment of hypothermia (lowered body temperature).

• Test your reactions to various nonprescription medications for motion sickness, which can be overwhelming in rough water.

• Practice the procedures for relieving cramps in deep water—you should knead and rub the affected muscle. Cramps can be very painful and devastating to a swimmer. Your hands, feet,

and calves are especially susceptible to cramping problems. Warm up and stretch out before you swim.

• Try using Vaseline to prevent chafing under your armpits and wherever your swimsuit might rub you, such as around your legs or under the shoulder straps.

• If you are going to swim for more than two hours, consider using high-calorie liquid supplements during your swim. This requires coordination with an assistant in an escort boat.

• If you will be accompanied by an escort boat, practice in advance so that you can stay with the boat as you swim.

• Practice looking forward periodically as you swim. You have to be able to sight landmarks to maintain your direction (there's no lane line on the bottom!).

• Learn to tread water with your legs only so that you'll be able to clear your goggles if they fill with water.

• Practice different breathing patterns (breathe every second, third, fourth, or fifth stroke). You may have to skip a breath every now and then if choppy waves are breaking over your head or if you're swimming in a group.

• You should be able to breathe to either side (alternate-side breathing) in crawl. This will equalize stress on both sides and permit you to breathe away from the waves if necessary.

• Though crawl stroke is best for most people, you may want to change strokes occasionally as a short break in a long swim.

Sometimes you'll actually have to enter a race to do an open-water swim. Experience will improve your performance if you learn from your mistakes and successes.

Consider the following additional advice, especially if you've never been in a race before:

• Although 75 to 85 percent of your training should be long-distance swimming, it's very easy to accommodate to this type of exercise by swimming very slowly. Be sure to spend some of your training time doing intervals and sprints to give you the reserve of power you may need in a race.

• Most distance swimmers do not emphasize the kick in their stroke, using the kick more for body position and balance than for great propulsion. Do some specific kicking drills in your workouts (5 to 10 percent), but don't overdo it.

• The start of the race is likely to be hectic, with the fastest swimmers jockeying for position and trying to find open space to swim in. Be prepared for this or you'll be off to a very bad start.

• A trained observer can count your strokes per minute, and this is the best standard of whether you're swimming at the right pace, swimming too slowly, or trying too hard. Normal references, such as speed per 50 or 100 yards, do not apply under these circumstances.

• You must go through the official finishing point and check yourself out of the race when you're done. Race officials must have everyone accounted for—either dropped out or finished—in the interest of safety.

• Don't get carried away with fantasies of winning and setting records. The two basic goals are to complete the event and to feel good about yourself afterwards.

EIGHT

Swimming Strokes

BASIC PROFICIENCY in several swimming strokes permits you to add variety to your training program. The basic fitness-swimming strokes are the crawl, back stroke, breast stroke, and elementary back stroke. Most fitness swimmers will be able to do these strokes. Although your swimming skills should be good, remember that you don't need to be a championship-level swimmer to get exercise benefits from fitness swimming.

This chapter, although it should be helpful to you, is not intended to be an exhaustive treatment of swimming technique. Study the illustrations and descriptions in terms of the hand and arm movements, foot and leg movements, method of breathing, and the coordination of the entire stroke. Practice each stroke in its parts—pulling and kicking—as well as the entire stroke. Work on the breathing pattern, too.

A swimming coach, lifeguard, competitive swimmer, or water safety instructor can check your strokes for you. Ask for one or two suggestions or corrections to work on for each stroke. Concentrate on these improvements each time you swim.

Some of you will do the butterfly in addition to the four basic strokes listed above, but most fitness swimmers do not use this stroke. It's not really part of our basic Fitness Swimming Course here at Dickinson College, but I do teach this stroke to individuals upon request. The difficulty of this stroke is greatly exaggerated. Thinking about it is a whole lot worse than actually doing it. It is most important to learn the butterfly stroke at a slow pace. Swim the stroke initially over very short distances so that you can maintain stroke rhythm and technique. Use a slow hand speed to feel yourself move forward through the water as your hands and arms move back. Keep your kick going, and breathe every second stroke. Do not swim to exhaustion—rest frequently, and build up very gradually. If you do just a little butterfly each time you swim, you will be amazed at how quickly you can develop this stroke.

Let's start, though, with refining the basic fitness-swimming strokes.

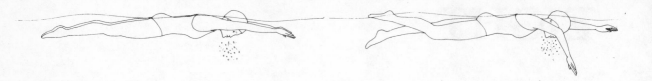

Crawl Stroke

PULLING ACTION. The hand enters the water fingertips first in front of the shoulder, with a small bend in the elbow creating a slight angle of entry with the hand and forearm. The entire arm-and-shoulder structure moves upward to achieve maximum stretch and reach during this hand entry position.

The hand moves down and back under the elbow just before a strong movement of the shoulder joint pulls the arm backward. In this "high-elbow position" underwater, the hand is directly beneath the elbow, and both the hand and forearm stay perpendicular to the water surface for as long as possible throughout the underwater pull. You should sense water pressure against your forearms during this propulsive part of the stroke.

During the single-arm pull, the upper arm and elbow point out away from the side of the body, and the amount of bend in the elbow varies throughout the underwater part of the stroke. The hand and forearm roughly point down toward the bottom of the pool throughout the underwater pull.

At the completion of the underwater pull, the palm of the hand turns to face the hip, and the hand moves upward and sideward into the recovery, with the little finger leaving the water first. The elbow bends to create a different high-elbow position over the surface of the water as the arm returns to the entry position.

KICKING ACTION. The legs alternate in the kicking action as the feet move up and down. The toes should be pointed, and the knees should bend and extend with emphasis on kicking backward and downward. The depth of the kick might be from 8 to 15 inches in a vertical plane.

The splashing action of the feet is caused by the heels just barely breaking the surface of the water, and this promotes a level body position in the stroke. The feet should not be lifted up above the water's surface.

BREATHING PATTERN. See Chapter 4 for full descriptions and learning tips on crawl stroke breathing patterns, which are covered there in great detail.

In brief, when the hand and arm move backward underwater and become even with the shoulder, turn to that side to

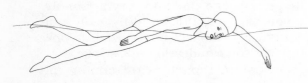

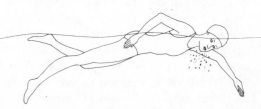

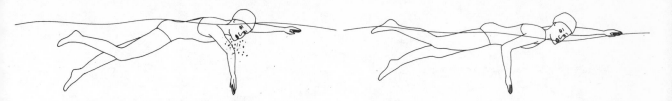

breathe. This pattern allows the breathing to be completed in time for the recovery of the arm. When the arm moves over the surface of the water, the face turns back down into the water at the same time, and you should look at the pool bottom about 2 to 4 feet in front of you. Do not always look toward the end of the pool as you swim. When properly done, movements of the hands, arms, shoulders, neck, and head all blend together into one smooth action.

Experiment frequently with the many different breathing patterns that can be used in the crawl stroke.

STROKE COORDINATION. The hand action is alternating: When one arm pulls, the other arm recovers. The hand action should be continuous, with the hand speed accelerating throughout the underwater pull. This momentum is then redirected into the over-the-surface recovery.

For most swimmers, the pull is relatively more important than the kick. Keep your feet moving, but set the rhythm of the stroke primarily with the hands and arms. The kick contributes

some to propulsion but helps mostly to maintain body position. Don't worry too much about the number of kicks per arm cycle. Usually, 4- to 6-beat kicks are sufficient for fitness swimming.

Though you remain horizontal from head to foot as you move through the water, there is considerable shoulder turning (rotation around the long axis of the body). That is, when the right arm is up in the recovery, the right shoulder is visible above the water surface; at the same time, the left arm is pulling underwater, and the left shoulder is down beneath the water surface. And vice versa. In other words, don't swim flat from side to side; turn onto your sides, as much as 40 to 50 degrees. The shoulders should turn or roll in coordination with the pulling, the recovery, and the breathing.

These shoulder-turning movements contribute to the momentum and reach of the arm stroke, permit you to move with less effort and muscular tension, and reflect a freedom of motion in the recovery characteristic of good swimmers. Body roll makes the recovery easier and the underwater pull stronger.

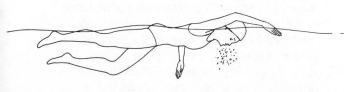

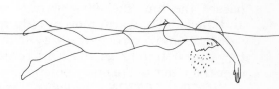

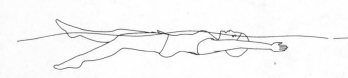

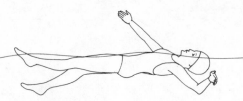

Back Stroke

PULLING ACTION. The hand enters the water just slightly outside the width of the shoulders, with the arm straight and the hand turned so that its little finger edge goes into the water first. The entire arm-and-shoulder structure moves upward to achieve maximum stretch and reach during this hand entry position.

At the start of the underwater pull, the hand moves out to the side and even with the elbow (modification of the high-elbow position). The hand and arm are pulled through by means of a strong shoulder-joint movement. Both the hand and forearm stay perpendicular to the midline of the body for as long as possible throughout the underwater pull.

The elbow is bent (as much as 90 degrees) during this propulsive action, and this single-arm pull is done with the hand 8 to 20 inches beneath the water surface, with the hand moving somewhat parallel to the surface of the water. The hand and forearm roughly point out toward the side of the pool throughout the underwater pull.

As the pull is completed and the hand passes the hip, the elbow straightens and the hand and arm move up (thumb-side first) into a vertical recovery. The elbow stays straight as the arm returns over the water to the entry position.

KICKING ACTION. The legs alternate in the kicking action as the feet move up and down. The toes should be pointed, and the knees should bend and extend with emphasis on kicking backward and upward. The depth of the kick might be from 8 to 15 inches in a vertical plane.

Neither the knees nor the feet should be lifted above the water surface. Concentrate on splashing the feet just slightly to ensure a level body position.

BREATHING PATTERN. Because your face is above the water surface, you can breathe in through the mouth whenever you wish; you should do this on a regular cycle, however. Exhale through the nose (some from the mouth) whenever you're not inhaling.

During the recovery, the arm may splash a small amount of water in your face, which can be very upsetting to a beginning swimmer. Using goggles and exhaling through your nose can help. In time, as you continue to practice this stroke, you'll become less sensitive to this problem.

STROKE COORDINATION. Head and body position are very important. Keep your chin up in a normal position, the back of your head in the water (not head back), your ears underwater, and both your chest and stomach up. Look straight up at the ceiling, don't move your head around, and kick up. Don't sit in the water. If your chin is down, the hips are too low, or the feet are too deep, your body position gets distorted away from a flat, horizontal position.

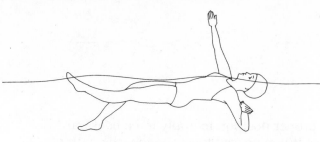

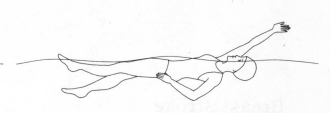

The hand action is alternating: When one arm pulls, the other arm recovers. The hand action should be continuous, with the hand speed accelerating throughout the underwater pull. This momentum is then redirected into the over-the-surface recovery. Don't make the common mistake of stopping the hand by your leg after each underwater pull. This results in uneven propulsion and destroys the continuous nature of the hand and arm action.

For most swimmers, the pull is relatively more important than the kick. Keep your feet moving, but set the rhythm of the stroke primarily with the hands and arms. The kick contributes some to propulsion but helps mostly to maintain body position. Don't worry too much about the number of kicks per arm cycle. Usually, 4- to 6-beat kicks are sufficient for fitness swimming.

Though you remain horizontal from head to foot as you move through the water, there is considerable shoulder turning (rotation around the long axis of the body). That is, when the right arm is up high in the recovery, the right shoulder is visible above the water surface; at the same time, the left arm is pulling underwater, and the left shoulder is down beneath the water surface. And vice versa. In other words, don't swim flat from side to side; turn onto your sides, as much as 40 to 50 degrees. The shoulders should turn or roll in coordination with the pulling and the recovery.

These shoulder-turning movements contribute to the momentum and reach of the arm stroke and permit you to move with less effort and muscular tension. What's more, they reflect a freedom of motion in the recovery characteristic of good swimmers. Body roll makes the recovery easier and the underwater pull stronger.

Some swimmers dislike the back stroke because they get disoriented while swimming on the back—they feel unsure of themselves because they seem to be upside down going backward. To deal with this problem, you might try taking short breaks to reorient yourself, periodically moving to a vertical position in the water. Continued practice, however, will enable you to become accustomed to the stroke, and it will no longer seem awkward.

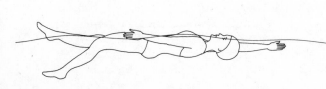

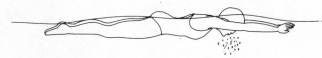

Breast Stroke

PULLING ACTION. In the starting position, the hands reach forward side by side just beneath the water surface, with the arms fully extended. The entire arm-and-shoulder structure moves upward to achieve maximum reach.

The hands separate, moving out to the side and down to create the high-elbow position in this stroke. The path of the hands is quite wide before the hands circle in under the face. The elbows move down under the shoulders and then continue forward (do not bring the upper arms and elbows back beyond shoulder level), and the hands reach forward in the underwater recovery of the arms back to the starting position.

KICKING ACTION. The starting position for the kick is with the legs fully extended near the surface of the water. The main objective is to push backward with the bottoms of the feet and the inside edges of the feet and ankles.

The knees bend considerably, and the hips bend slightly, to recover the feet up near the buttocks. The knees should be a hand's width apart or just slightly more. Do not spread them too far apart and point them out to the sides or hold them tightly together. The upper legs and knees should point down at the bottom of the pool. Hook the feet (draw up the toes toward the shins), and then turn them outward. The feet at this point are wider apart than the knees. All these movements are simply to get the feet in

proper position to apply force backward.

When viewed from the top, the path of the feet in the propulsive part of this kick is slightly out, back, and then together in a long, flat curve. When viewed from the side, the path of the feet is primarily in a horizontal plane, although the feet may finish just a little lower than their starting point in this propulsive action. Propulsion results from strong extension movements of the knees and hips.

Just before the feet come together at the completion of the kick, as they return to the starting position, the soles turn inward to face each other. The recovery of the legs (bending the knees and turning the feet out) should be done somewhat slower than the propulsive action (pushing backward with the feet). When these movements are performed at the same speed, they tend to cancel each other out, and you will have very little forward progress.

BREATHING PATTERN. Lift your head and begin to breathe to the front when the hands are wide in the high-elbow position. Complete the breathing as the elbows move below the shoulders; continue forward without pausing.

There is thus a natural link between the downward action of the arms and the lift to the front for the breath, and the

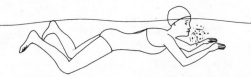

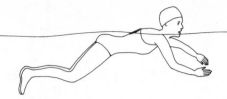

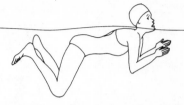

arm action and the breathing blend together so well that no hesitation or hitch in the arm stroke is necessary to complete the breathing. After the breath, the face goes back down into the water as the hands go forward to a fully stretched-out position. Look down at the bottom of the pool at this point, about 2 or 3 feet in front of you. Do not look at the other end of the pool as you glide forward.

It seems to fit the rhythm of this stroke best to breathe on every stroke. There are natural up-and-down movements as you swim this stroke, resulting from the alternation between the elbows-down, head-up position and the hands-forward, head-down, look-down position.

STROKE COORDINATION. The basic coordination of this stroke is as follows: first you pull and breathe, then you kick, then you stretch out and glide.

The relative contributions of the pull and the kick are more equal in this stroke than in the crawl, back stroke, and butterfly stroke, and for many swimmers, power is split about 50-50 between the pull and the kick. Some breast strokers are arm-oriented, however, while others have stronger legs.

A primary objective in this stroke is to create as smooth a transition of power as possible from your arms to your legs. If you pull back too far beyond the shoulders, you'll tend to stop the hands and destroy the rhythm of the stroke. If you breathe too late, you'll interrupt the flow of the short, wide, circular, continuous hand action.

A maximum reach forward with the hands is very important because it gives the feet a chance to finish the kick, contributing more to the total propulsion. If the hands go forward and then immediately separate to start the next stroke, the swimmer will be beset with problems: weakened arm action because of the forward momentum created by the kick, a tendency to pull too far back beyond the shoulders, mistiming of the breathing pattern, and a running together of the pull and the kick. This phase of the stroke has often been described as a brief glide or ride forward, and you should stretch out as you reach your hands all the way forward, in a position similar to hanging from a chinning bar, while looking at your hands, which are close together.

One of the challenges of this stroke is to reduce to a minimum the periods of sudden deceleration that follow the periods of acceleration, in order to create more even and efficient movement through the water.

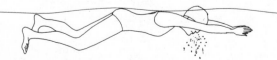

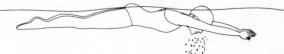

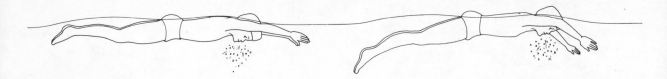

Butterfly Stroke

PULLING ACTION. The hands enter the water at shoulder width or a little wider, with a slight bend in the elbows. The entire arm-and-shoulder structure moves upward to achieve maximum stretch and reach during this hand entry position.

The hands move down and back under the elbows just before strong movements of the shoulder joints pull the arms backward. In this high-elbow position underwater, the hands are directly beneath the elbows, and both the hands and forearms stay perpendicular to the water surface for as long as possible throughout the underwater pull. You should sense water pressure against your hands and forearms during this propulsive arm stroke.

During the double-arm pull, the upper arms and elbows point out away from the sides of the body, and the distance between the hands varies with the amount of bend in the elbows at different points in the underwater stroke. The hands and forearms roughly point down toward the bottom of the pool throughout the underwater pull.

Just before finishing the underwater stroke, the hands may move slightly closer to each other before swinging outward and upward into the recovery. At the completion of the underwater pull, the palms turn toward the hips, and the hands move upward and sideward into the recovery, with the little fingers leaving the water first. The hands recover just over and somewhat parallel to the surface of the water, with the palms down or facing the surface. Although the recovery is wide, the elbows bend slightly as the hands return to the entry position.

KICKING ACTION. Both feet and legs move up and down at the same time, and the knees bend and extend; the emphasis is on kicking down and back in a vertical plane with the feet and toes pointed. Skilled swimmers will also have an upkick as the straight legs return to the surface in preparation for the next kick.

The heels will cause some splashing as they break the water surface at the completion and start of each kick. There is an undulating action to this dolphin kick, and the hips move up and down in reaction to the movements of the feet and legs.

BREATHING PATTERN. As the hands and arms move backward underwater and become even with the shoulders, lift your head to breathe. Lift your head only

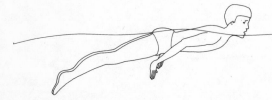

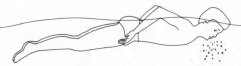

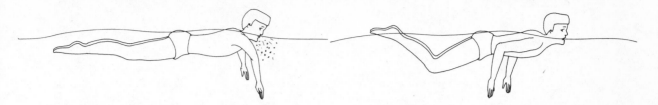

high enough to get a breath (put your chin on the surface of the water), and look forward during the breathing.

In general, you should breathe every second stroke in order to distort the body position the least and to fit the rhythm of this stroke the best. With this pattern, the breathing is completed in time for the recovery of the hands and arms. As the hands go forward, the head should go back down into the water but should stay within the area formed by the chest and shoulders. Look at the pool bottom about 2 to 4 feet in front of you; do not always look at the end of the pool as you swim.

It is also possible to breathe to the side in the butterfly stroke. This is much less common than front breathing because it tends to distort the swimmer's body position, but some swimmers have been very successful with this variation.

STROKE COORDINATION. The hand action should be continuous; do not stop the hands at their entry into or exit from the water. Hand speed varies, however, and the hands accelerate as they move backward against the water. Every swimmer has an optimum hand speed, and overstroking (moving the hands too fast or too hard) causes the hands to slip through the water without good contact, much like the spinning of a car's wheels.

Usually there are two dolphin kicks per arm cycle—one as the hands enter the water and one at the completion of the underwater pull. A few good swimmers use just one kick, and many show a major kick followed by a minor, or trail, kick. Any of these patterns is acceptable, especially for fitness swimmers. Try to keep your feet moving.

The hands move at the same time and the feet move at the same time. But set the rhythm of this stroke primarily with the hands and arms, and then let the kick fit into that stroke rhythm.

When properly done, the breathing pattern and the hand action should blend together very smoothly. As the hands pull back, the head lifts forward to breathe. As the hands recover forward, the head goes back down into the water. Breathing too late causes problems such as stopping the hands at the end of the underwater pull, inability to fit the kicks into the arm action, and incoordination in the entire stroke.

Although the body position is flat from side to side, there are substantial up-and-down movements of the shoulders, trunk, and hips as the swimmer moves forward through the water in an undulating pattern.

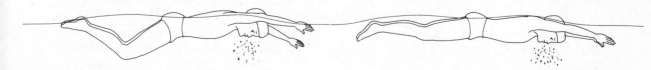

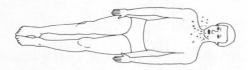

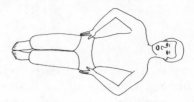

Elementary Back Stroke

PULLING ACTION. The hand and arm action in this stroke can be simply described as up-out-together. From the starting, gliding position by the sides of the legs, the hands recover up the sides of the body and then outward slightly above shoulder level.

The propulsive action is a double-arm pull, with the elbows slightly bent and the hands moving parallel to the water surface at a depth of 4 to 8 inches. Keep your hands and forearms perpendicular to the midline of the body for as long as possible during this underwater pull.

As the pull is completed and your hands pass the hips, the elbows straighten in a definite push and the hands return to the starting, gliding position with the palms facing the sides of the legs.

KICKING ACTION. The starting, gliding position for the kick is with the legs fully extended near the surface of the water. The main objective is to propel yourself backward with the bottoms of the feet and the inside edges of the feet and ankles.

To perform the kick, bend the knees about 90 degrees, dropping the feet be-neath the knees. The knees should be a hand's width apart or just slightly more. Do not spread them too far apart and point them out to the sides or hold them tightly together. The upper legs and knees should point toward the end wall of the pool. Do not lift them above the water surface. Hook the feet (draw up the toes toward the shins), and then turn them outward. The feet at this point are wider apart than the knees. All these movements are simply to get the feet in position to apply force backward.

When viewed from the top, the path of the feet in the propulsive part of this kick is slightly out, back, and then together in a long, flat curve. When viewed from the side, the path of the feet is primarily upward to the surface. Propulsion results from strong extension movements of the knees.

Just before the feet come together at the completion of the kick, as they return to the starting, gliding position, the soles turn inward to face each other. The recovery of the legs (bending the knees and turning the feet out) should be done somewhat slower than the propulsive action (pushing backward with the feet). When these movements are performed

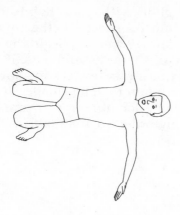

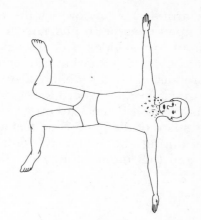

at the same speed, they tend to cancel each other out, and you will have very little forward progress.

BREATHING PATTERN. Because your face is above the water surface, you can breathe in through the mouth whenever you wish; you should do this on a regular cycle, however. Exhale through the nose (some from the mouth) whenever you're not inhaling.

For most swimmers, a natural pattern is to breathe in during the recovery phase and out during the propulsive phase of this stroke.

STROKE COORDINATION. Head and body position are very important. Keep your chin up in a normal position, the back of your head in the water (not head

back), your ears underwater, and both your chest and stomach up. Look straight up at the ceiling, don't move your head around, and kick up and back. Don't sit in the water. If your chin is down, the hips are too low, or the feet are too deep, your body position gets distorted away from a flat, horizontal position.

The arm and leg recoveries occur at the same time, as do their propulsive movements. The feet may finish the kick just before the hands finish the pull, because the feet move through slightly less distance than the hands do. The hands, feet, and knees should remain underwater, and there should be no splashing in this stroke.

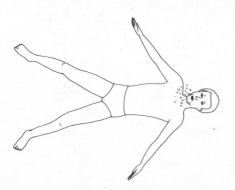

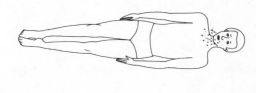

The arm and leg recoveries (from the arms-up, knees-bent position to the arms out to the sides, feet turned out) should be done somewhat slower than the propulsive action (double-arm pull, outward-backward-upward kick), or you will have very little forward progress.

The speed of the hands and feet accelerates during the propulsive pull and kick, and this momentum runs into a short glide with your hands by your sides and your feet together. When the glide slows down, you begin the next recovery of the arms and legs. If you are using this stroke as a resting stroke, you can maintain the glide longer. If you are swimming for fitness, you can use less glide in order to maintain more even propulsion.

NINE

Turns and Push-offs

AFTER PERFORMING A TURN and pushing off from the pool wall, most fitness swimmers immediately start to swim. Good swimmers, however, never swim between the wall and the back stroke flags (also the point where the surface lane lines change from a solid color to alternating colors). Instead, they glide in a streamlined position, catching a free ride for the first 5 yards of each length. You could swim for your entire lifetime and never swim faster than the speed of your push-off. A good push-off gives you lots of momentum and speed going into each length.

The heart of every turn is a strong push and glide. Push hard with your knees, ankles, and feet. Face-up or face-down, you should be able to push off and then glide at least 15 feet.

To push off on your front, start slightly underwater with your face down, push with your legs, and glide gradually to the surface. Stretch out from your fingertips down through your toes. Keep your hands together, your arms overhead, and your head squeezed between your arms.

To push off on your back, push off with your hands by your sides and your face up. You don't need to go underwater on this type of simple back push-off.

Study the illustrations and brief descriptions to get the key parts of each of the turns. Try to have your turns checked by a swimming coach or competitive swimmer who can give you some corrections or suggestions. In addition to the turns and push-offs performed throughout your workouts, you can also practice these skills in special sessions at the start or finish of your workouts. Don't swim a lot in this special practice—just work from a stroke or two beyond the flags into the wall and then back out.

In the stroke turns, you'll use the same stroke coming into and going out from the wall. In the changing turns (also called transition turns), you'll change strokes at the wall—for example, from crawl to back, back to breast, and breast to elementary back in the fitness medley. Once you get these turns down, you'll be able to switch easily from one stroke to any other.

CRAWL STROKE TURN

1. Swim in to a one-hand touch.
2. Tuck up and swing your feet in to the wall. Breathe in as you turn around.
3. Bring one arm over and go underwater slightly. Exhale through your nose.
4. Bring your hands together, turn your face down, and execute a strong leg push.
5. Glide in a streamlined position on your front.
6. Start two or three kicks.
7. Pull with one arm, then stroke with the other arm and breathe.

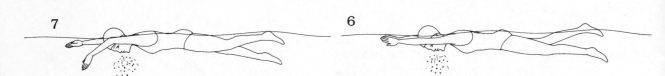

BACK STROKE TURN

1. Swim in to a one-hand touch.
2. Turn over toward that hand.
3. Tuck up and swing your feet in to the wall. Breathe in as you turn around.
4. Gently place the back of your head on the surface of the water. Release your hands from the wall.
5. Put your hands by your sides and execute a strong leg push. Keep your face up, and exhale through your nose. You don't need to go underwater on this turn.
6. Glide in a streamlined position on your back.
7. Start two or three kicks.
8. Start one arm up and over, then the other.

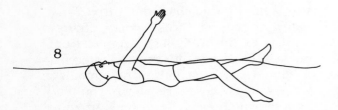
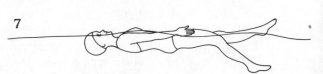

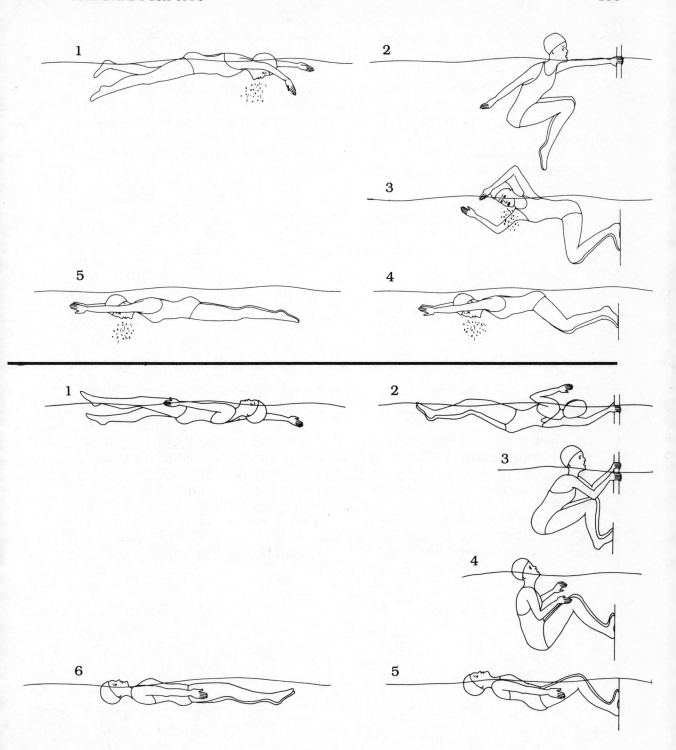

BREAST STROKE TURN

1. Swim in to a two-hand touch.
2. Tuck up and swing your feet in to the wall. Breathe in as you turn around.
3. Bring one arm over and go underwater slightly. Exhale through your nose.
4. Bring your hands together, turn your face down, and execute a strong leg push.

5. Glide in a streamlined position on your front.
6. Start the arm stroke for breast stroke.
7. Lift your head to breathe during the arm pull.
8. Finish your kick. Put your face down in the water as you reach forward, with a short glide before your next arm stroke.

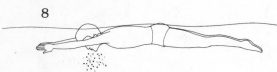 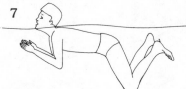 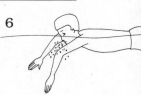

ELEMENTARY BACK STROKE TURN

1. Swim in to a one-hand touch.
2. Turn over toward that hand.
3. Tuck up and swing your feet in to the wall. Breathe in as you turn around.
4. Gently place the back of your head on the surface of the water. Release your hands from the wall.

5. Put your hands by your sides and execute a strong leg push. Keep your face up, and exhale through your nose. You don't need to go underwater on this turn.
6. Glide in a streamlined position on your back.
7. Start the regular stroke again.

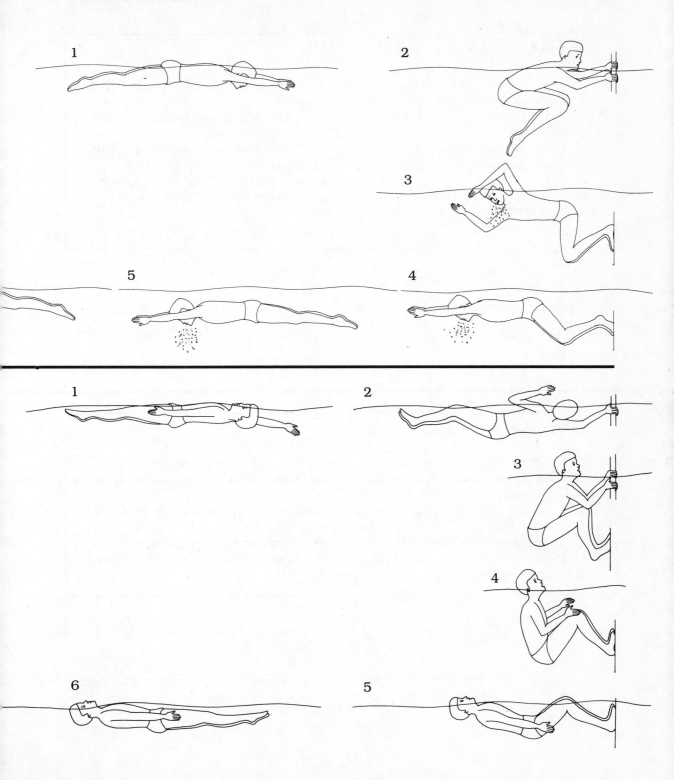

BUTTERFLY TURN

1. Swim in to a two-hand touch.
2. Tuck up and swing your feet in to the wall. Breathe in as you turn around.
3. Bring one arm over and go underwater slightly. Exhale through your nose.
4. Bring your hands together, turn your face down, and execute a strong leg push.

5. Glide in a streamlined position on your front.
6. Begin one or two kicks.
7. Finish first dolphin kick.
8. Begin and finish second dolphin kick. Start the butterfly arm pull. Take one pull with your face down, and then breathe during the next arm stroke.

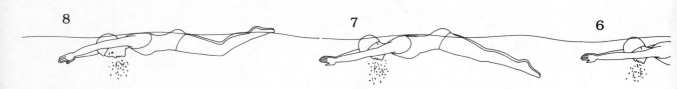

CRAWL-TO-BACK TURN

1. Swim in to a two-hand touch.
2. Tuck up and swing your feet in to the wall. Breathe in as you turn.
3. Gently place the back of your head on the surface of the water. Release your hands from the wall.
4. Put your hands by your sides, and execute a strong leg push. Keep your face up, and exhale through your nose. You don't need to go underwater on this turn.
5. Glide in a streamlined position on your back.
6. Start two or three kicks.
7. Start one arm up and over, then the other.

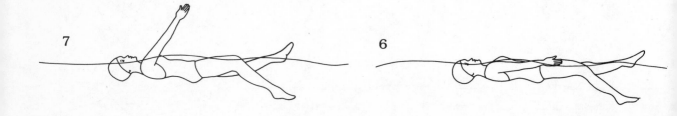

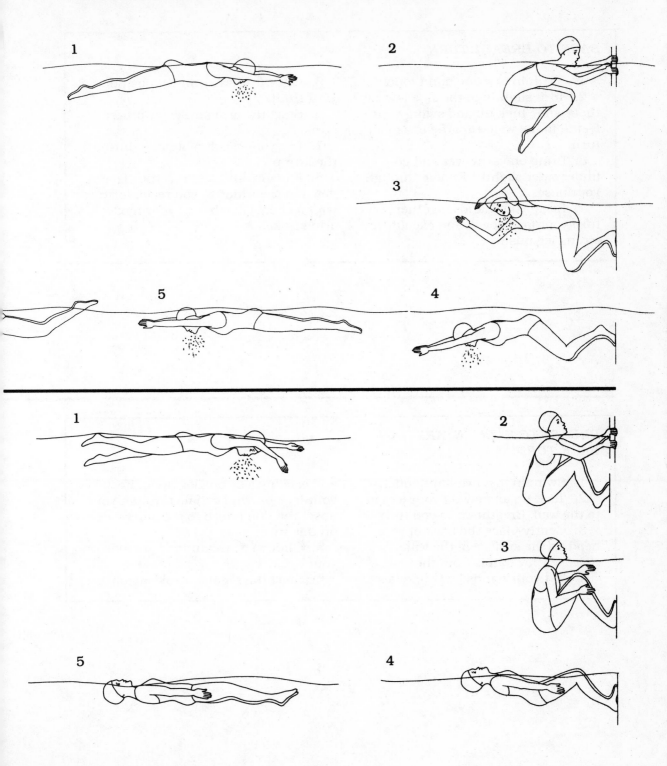

BACK-TO-BREAST TURN

1. Swim in to a one-hand touch.
2. Turn slightly to the side toward that hand. Tuck up and swing your feet in to the wall. Breathe in as you turn.
3. Bring one arm over and go underwater slightly. Exhale through your nose.
4. Bring your hands together, turn your face down, and execute a strong leg push.

5. Glide in a streamlined position on your front.
6. Start the arm stroke for breast stroke.
7. Lift your head to breathe during the arm pull.
8. Finish your kick. Put your face down in the water as you reach forward, with a short glide before your next arm stroke.

8 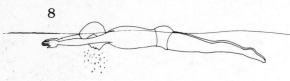   7 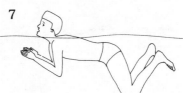   6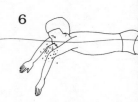

BREAST-TO-ELEMENTARY BACK TURN

1. Swim in to a two-hand touch.
2. Tuck up and swing your feet in to the wall. Breathe in as you turn.
3. Gently place the back of your head on the surface of the water. Release your hands from the wall.
4. Put your hands by your sides and execute a strong leg push. Keep your face up, and exhale through your nose. You don't need to go underwater on this turn.

5. Glide in a streamlined position on your back.
6. Start the regular stroke again.

6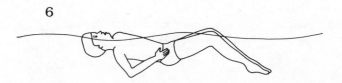

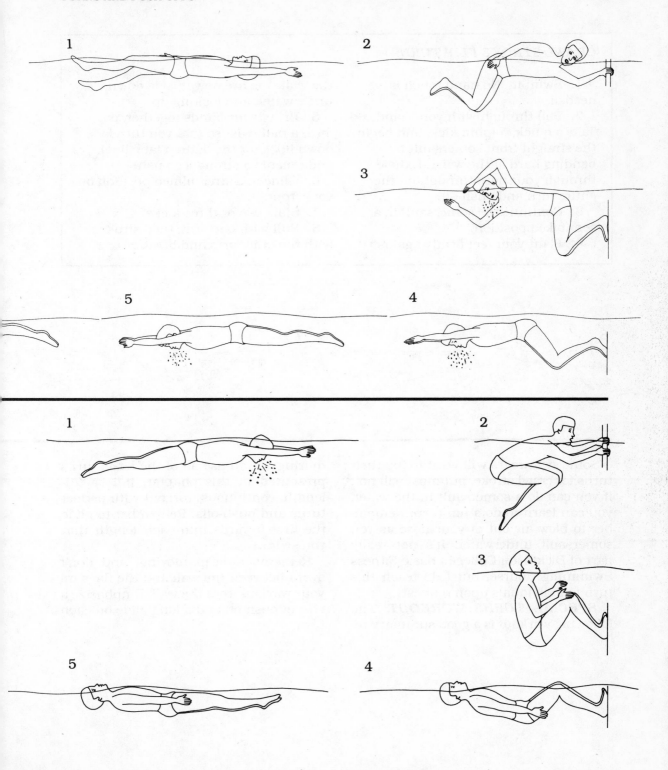

CRAWL STROKE FLIP TURN

1. Swim in. No hand touch is needed.

2. Pull through with your hands. Take a quick dolphin kick, and begin the straight front somersault by bending hard at the waist. Exhale through your nose throughout the entire turn and push-off.

3. Continue the somersault in a semipiked position.

4. Plant your feet firmly against the wall. You are now upside down, underwater, and looking up.

5. Bring your hands together, perform a half twist so that you turn face down (look for the bottom lane line), and execute a strong leg push.

6. Glide in a streamlined position on your front.

7. Start two or three kicks.

8. Pull with one arm, then stroke with the other arm and breathe.

8

7

Some swimmers will want to flip their turns for crawl stroke, but most will not. If you can do a somersault in the water, you can learn to do a flip turn. Remember to blow air out of your nose as you somersault underwater. It's not really part of Dickinson College's basic Fitness Swimming Course, but I do teach this turn to individuals upon request.

SPECIAL TURNS WORKOUT. The following workout is a good summary re-quiring you to use all of the basic turns presented in this chapter. It is a 20-length, continuous workout with perfect turns and push-offs. Remember to glide the first 5 yards into each length that you swim.

Remember, keep moving, and don't swim between the wall and the flags on your way out from the wall. Emphasize a strong push-off and a long glide on each turn.

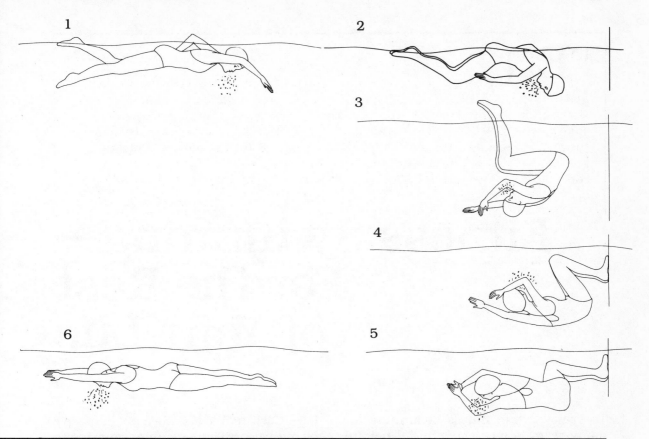

WORKOUT 202

	Dates Completed		
2 lengths crawl			
2 lengths back			
2 lengths breast			
2 lengths elementary back			
8 lengths repeating above strokes in reverse order			
1 length crawl			
1 length back			
1 length breast			
1 length elementary back			
20 total			

TEN

Fitness Swimming—
For the Rest
of Your Life

To STAY ACTIVE in fitness swimming for many years, some people find it helpful to have swimming challenges or the support of a group. This chapter may provide a loose network for this type of support. You can participate in some of these activities from a distance, or you may be able to adapt them for use by a local pool.

FITNESS SWIMMING CLUB. Induction into this club follows the completion of 100 miles (7,040 lengths) of fitness-swimming workouts. This one-time-only membership requirement is a realistic one-year project for most regular fitness swimmers. If you would like to join, keep track of your swimming distances in a daily log. Once you have completed 100 miles, submit your log to Fitness Swimming Club, Kline Center, Dickinson College, Carlisle, PA 17013. You will receive by mail a certificate verifying your membership.

WORKOUT OF THE WEEK. Every Monday at our pool, a new fitness-swimming workout of the week is posted. Each week, different formats are used and different distances are called for. This procedure adds variety and challenge to the workouts of the fitness swimmers who choose to try it, encouraging them to follow a planned and structured workout and try new strokes and sets and subsets. Occasionally one of our regular swimmers prepares the fitness workout of the week. If you're traveling in this area, please plan to stop in and try the posted workout. Please call in advance of your arrival to arrange the details.

FITNESS SWIMMING HOTLINE. The Fitness Swimming Hotline has been established in our office to answer your questions or to talk about any aspect of your fitness-swimming program. A swim coach or instructor is usually available between 9 A.M. and 3 P.M., Monday through Friday, depending on classes, meetings, and travel schedule. If no one is here, leave your name and number and we'll return your call.

The exercise dropout rate is higher if you're doing this all by yourself. It's easy to get discouraged, especially at the beginning, if no one can answer your questions or help you with your problems. Please feel free to call. The hotline number is (717) 245-1523.

SPECIAL AWARDS. In addition to the 100-mile club, Dickinson College sponsors several other fitness-swimming awards. I hope these awards will provide some incentive for you to stick with fitness swimming for a long time. If you complete any of the challenges, submit a letter recording your achievement, the date of completion, and the details of your swim. You will receive by mail a certificate that verifies your performance.

• *Super Swims.* Super Swims are long, continuous swims with no equipment. To complete them, fitness swimmers, on a one-time basis, swim longer and farther than they normally would in their daily workouts. Doing an extra-long workout is a great way to end a school semester or a half-year or year of fitness swimming. There are four distances of Super Swims: 2,500 yards (100 lengths), 3,000 yards (120 lengths), 4,000 yards (160 lengths), and 5,000 yards (200 lengths).

• *200 Miles in One Year Award.* For the 200 Miles in One Year Award, you must average approximately 1,000 yards (40 lengths) per day throughout the entire year. You could achieve this distance by swimming one mile four times a week for fifty weeks. Use a daily log to keep track of your actual distances in each workout.

• *1,000-Mile Club.* You'll need a multiyear commitment to swim far enough to qualify for the 1,000-Mile Club. There's no time limit. Just keep track of your mileage with detailed and cumulative written records.

• *1,000,000-Yard Club.* The 1,000,000-Yard Club is actually an intermediate step on the way to the 1,000 miles. One million yards equals 568.18 miles. This should provide some encouragement as you get past the halfway point in your 1,000-mile goal. Here again, use a daily log to chart your swimming distances.

BEYOND FITNESS SWIMMING. During the past twelve years here at Dickinson College, most of our physical education staff have been refining our required physical education program into a new curriculum concept called Truly Living—Dickinson's Program for Lifestyle Enhancement. It has become a model program that will carry us well past the year 2000. This program tries to offset the students' likely lack of education about how to live as physical and emotional beings, and to help them understand that their bad habits are probably regarded as normal by their friends and by society as a whole. Although designed for a small liberal arts college, Truly Living could be modified for elementary schools, high schools, other types of colleges or universities, or corporations. Most important, it could provide guidelines and directions to help you as an individual to create a healthier lifestyle.

I especially want you to understand that there is more to wellness than just physical fitness, and I hope you will go beyond the scope of this book to explore various aspects of lifestyle management. Wellness programs take a proactive, holistic, and preventive approach to health care, with great emphasis on each individual's responsibility for his or her own well-being.

This book covers just one small but important part of all those things that we ought to know and ought to do to greatly improve the quality of our lives. I hope that you will be able to go beyond the contents of this book by finding a comparable program in your area—one that integrates health-related knowledge and wellness principles with lifetime sports and fitness activities. I also hope that you will participate in other fitness activities in addition to your continued involvement in fitness swimming and that you'll go beyond fitness swimming in a lifetime pursuit of "living well."

It's a great day
to take a swim!

Further Readings

OVER THE YEARS I've written several articles in the field of swimming for fitness. Reprints of the following are available upon request. Write to Fitness Swimming Club, Kline Center, Dickinson College, Carlisle, PA 17013.

"Fitness Swimming in Small Pools." *National Aquatics Journal* (Summer 1991): 15.

"Fitness Swimming: How to Teach It." *Aqua Notes—Newsletter of The AAHPERD Aquatics Council,* 8, no. 2 (September 1989): 4–5.

"Heads Up Workout." *The Finals—From the Top*, V 89-3 (July–September 1989): 4.

"Self-Paced Triathlon Course." *National Aquatics Journal* (Spring 1989): 7–9.

"Beyond Phys. Ed." *Dickinson Magazine* (October 1988): p. 27.

"Expand Your Workout Options for Fitness Swimming." *National Aquatics Journal* (Fall 1988): 2–3, 17.

"Teaching Fitness Swimming." *National Aquatics Journal* (Spring 1988): 7–10.

"Swimming for Time: Try These Short, Timed Workouts as a Stopgap." *SwimSwim Magazine* (Summer 1984): 20–21. This article also appeared in *Triathlon*, February 1985, 16–17.

"Fitness Swimming: Something Old, Something New." *GAHPER Journal* (Georgia) (Winter 1979): 12–13.

"Portrait of a Lifetime Swimmer: Dr. Loree Florence." *Swimmers Quarterly* (Sept.–Nov. 1978): 40–41.

Index